HIV/AIDS Among Industrial & Transport Workers

A Hand Book

Prof. Rajinder M. Kalra

Revised Version

To order additional copies of this book, contact:
Xlibris Corporation
0-800-644-6988
www.xlibrispublishing.co.uk
Orders@xlibrispublishing.co.uk
303512

2

Contributing Author (Hony) Dr. Rakesh Mehta MD, FRCPC FACIP Clinical Associate Professor New York Medical College

Contributing Author (Hony) Archana Uppal

Research Assistants (Volunteer Hony)

Rajan Brar

Nikki Brar

CONTENTS

Medical Consultants Manuscript Voluntary Contributions

The author is grateful to the following medical professionals for giving their views about this manuscript on voluntary basis.

- Dr. Rakesh Mehta MD, FRCPC FACIP is a Clinical Associate Professor, New York Medical College, New York.

- Dr. Virender Bhatti, M.D., General Physician, British Columbia, Canada.

- Dr. Asoke Dutt F.R.C.S Canada

- Dr. Hilda Stranger F.R.C.P. (C) F.A.C.C., British Columbia, Canada.

- Dr. George S. Athwal, M.D., F.R.C.S. (C), University of Western Ontario, St. Joseph's Hospital London, Ontario, Canada.

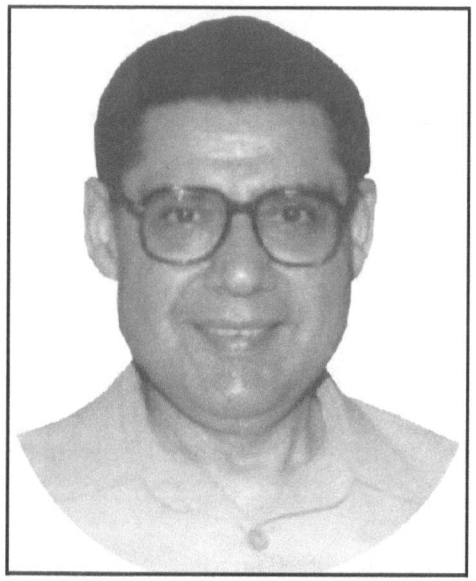

In Loving Memory of Mr. C.M. Chawla CMD Vikas Publishing House Delhi for his inspiration to the author concerning HIV/AIDS menace in the society.

ACKNOWLEDGEMENTS

The author expresses his gratitude to his wife Mrs. Santosh Kalra for assisting him in writing the manuscript. The author (Kalra) expresses his special gratitude to late Reverend Mother Teresa and his Holiness the Dalai Lama noble laureates for their inspiration in his academic and professional growth.

The author is also indebted to the following persons:

–Late Mr. C.M Chawla, CMD, Vikas Publishing House Private LTD. Delhi, India. For his valuable contributions and encouragement in this academic venture.

–Late Mrs. and Dr. P.C. Mehta for being a source of inspiration for the author.

–Special thanks to Mr. Piyush Chawla and Ms. Veena Baswani for their academic advice.

–Dr. Rakesh Mehta faculty member of New York Medical College, Valhalla, New York for his cooperation and encouragement.

–Col. Rajinder Datta (Transport Workers Submission) British Columbia, Canada.

PREFACE

India has emerged as a country with one of the largest number of citizens infected with HIV/AIDS. More than 3 million of India's 1 billion people are infected with HIV, the virus that leads to AIDS. The Government of India and numerous NGO's are focusing on AIDS prevention through media, social interaction and education.

The burden of disease, however is too great and much work needs to be done on prevention strategies, especially among industrial and transport workers.

Industrial workers are the backbone of our economy and nation builders. It is essential, therefore, that AIDS prevention education be an integral component during initiating and training of these workers in any industry.

HIV infection is an un-precedent challenge for today's highly advanced medical science. The curse has indiscriminately fallen on all sects of society sparing not even the new born child due to HIV infection in mother.

Despite the relentless struggle to check its spread and find a vaccine to control it, the success has been just enough to prolong the life of the affected person by administrating expensive cocktails of medicines. The Antiretroviral Therapy (ART) is not very easily available and affordable to the reach of the less fortunate people who form a vast majority of those suffering from the HIV infection. The Known certainty about the HIV is its mode of transmission which is:

(1.) Exchange of Body fluids of infected persons blood, serum, vaginal fluids or blood infected saliva.

(2.) New born baby of the infected mother from the mother's blood at the time of delivery or even the foetus may contract the infection in the womb.

Since sexual behavior mainly determines the exchange of body fluids, educating the public especially young people to modify their sexual behavior is imperative to control the HIV Epidemic.

Having sex with one known person who is free from the HIV infection is the safest way to avoid HIV/AIDS Epidemic but in our modern complex social patterns where young people have to wait far too long to establish permanent relationships because of economical and social reasons, sexual behavior in most societies today can vary from one night stands to casual sex with multiple partners or even homosexuality.

This scenario is further complicated with abuse of alcohol and drug addiction (I.V.)

Therefore, awareness and prevention programmes through education about HIV/AIDS Epidemic need to be a mandatory part of any training or orientation programme for youth development, employment and management.

Special attention needs to be given to the high risk groups:

- Sex Workers
- Migrant Workers
- Industrial Workers
- Truck Drivers
- Professionals engaged in handling blood products especially blood transfusion.
- Young persons who could be absolutely ignorant about the perils of indulging in unsafe sex, they could also be exploited by older men and women.

The focus of this handbook is on HIV/AIDS among Industrial workers and transport workers with special reference to India.

The author has already developed a hand book with American Authors (Prof. Francis X. Sutman and Ms. Archana Uppal) titled "World Perspective on HIV and AIDS Epidemic for less Fortunate".

The author of this hand book has suggested the establishment of effective counseling centres focusing on AIDS prevention, drug de-addiction and alcohol abuse in each and every industry unit.

Prof. Rajinder M. Kalra

INTRODUCTION

In a recent publication titled AIDS—No Time for Complacency, the World Health Organization warns that socio economic impact of HIV/AIDS threatens the very fabric of society. It affects people in their most productive age, resulting in direct and indirect economic costs—because AIDS incapacitates people at ages when they are most needed for the support of the young and the elderly, the impact on families—is enormous, and is aggravated by the frequent stigmatization of people with HIV/AIDS."

A UNAIDS press release (2006) mentioned that more than 40 million people worldwide are/living with HIV related diseases. The worst affected regions are the most populated regions of Africa, India, China Latin America, and the Caribbean. The poor people in many developing countries are worst affected because of illiteracy and poverty, use of narcotics, alcohol, unprotected sex and reckless sexual behaviour.

The HIV infection has been around for more than two decades and therefore the number of people dying with AIDS is going to Increase every year because those who contracted HIV virus ten years ago or even earlier have lived their expected period of survival.

About two decades ago HIV virus that causes AIDS was first recognized as a killer virus, a disease that to this day has no really effective and economically viable cure. Therefore, prevention is absolutely necessary to check the possible endemic spread of the virus.

The WHO (World Health Organization), UNAIDS, UNICEF, ILO, other international and national organizations spared no efforts to send warnings about this incurable virus/disease. The whole world became aware of the

HIV and AIDS Epidemic spreading in developed and developing countries indiscriminately. HIV is a global challenge and requires a global response. HIV/AIDS in the world of work needs intensive efforts to overcome this killer monster as it makes an enormous impact essentially in the industrial sector.

Industrial workers are the backbone of economy of any country and they are the nation builders. Therefore, it is essential that awareness and prevention of HIV/AIDS must be an important component during initiation and training of these industrial workers in any industry.

Coming to the specifics of Transport Industry, it is worth mentioning that Government and numerous NGO's such as International Transport Workers Federation (ITF) are making sincere efforts for bringing Awareness and Prevention of HIV/AIDS through media print, social interaction, seminars, workshops and thereby educating industrial workers especially the transport sector.

Global Preview—International Transport Workers Federation ITF: HIV/AIDS Awareness and Prevention

In the 1980's the ITF and some of its affiliates made valuable contributions in organizing programmes for different types of transport workers concerning HIV/AIDS Awareness and Prevention at the global level. These programmes are focused on sub-Saharan Africa, South Asia, India, Pakistan and other countries. The ITF has 666 affiliates in 142 countries. The mission of this organization is to initiate a battle against HIV/AIDS among transport workers all over the world through education concerning fear, stigma and discrimination against HIV positive person's awareness and prevention of HIV infection, safe sex, harmful effects of intravenous drug abuse, alcohol consumption and a healthy lifestyle.

Major Initiatives of ITF (International Transport Workers Federation

- HIV / AIDS and Transport Workers in Africa
- HIV / AIDS and Transport Workers—South Asia
- Seafarer's Health Information Program (SHIP)
- Joint Regional HIV/AIDS project in the Abidfour Lagos transport corridor.

- ITF has a meaningful collaboration with other global unions through E-Bulletins which are involved in the profile of "HIV and the Work peace.

HIV/AIDS in Africa

South Africa is in the midst of a HIV/AIDS crisis. More than 13% of the population is affected by HIV/AIDS.

Given this massive problem of HIV and Aids Epidemic and its impact on adults of prime working age, the threatening implication on economic and non-economic factors cane be catastrophic. It will slow down the rate of economic growth which is one of the major fallouts of HIV and AIDS Epidemic. HIV/AIDS is a real threat to development, economic growth and the elevation of poverty in Africa. The negative effects of HIV/AIDS facing the African continent are now being recognized and steps are being taken to address this menace. The exact death toll cannot be estimated as the AIDS Epidemic continues to spread and affect all regions of Africa.

In the Latin America and the Caribbean (LAC) region about 6,000 people have died from AIDS. Latin America had the highest number of new infections during 2005, totaling more than 200,000. The negative impact of injecting harmful drugs, unsafe sex, poverty, illiteracy, unemployment with stigma and discrimination of persons living with HIV and AIDS are some key challenges and issues concerning HIV infections in small countries like Argentina, Brazil, Chile, Guatemala and Honduras etc.

In Caribbean region HIV and AIDS Epidemic claimed 24,000 lives in 2005 (Age 15-44). A total of 300,000 people are living with HIV infection including the 30,000 who were newly HIV infected in 2005. There is a rising trend of HIV infection and lack of decent job opportunities.

The world of work response: Progress

The ILO (International Labour Organization) Code of practice on HIV/ Aids and the World of work was initiated in Argentina in 2003.

Workers and employers organizations are active partners in the 'Red Ribbon' campaign—Tripartite Body Agreement, the battle against HIV/AIDS is on the country's labour agenda.

In Chile, ILO and the National Copper Corporation has devised an internal plan based on the recommendations of ILO's practical recommendations concerning HIV/AIDS Epidemic.

UNAIDS, the World Economic Forum and ILO have initiated partnership development in Brazil, Jamaica and Honduras.

The Jamaica Employers Federation has signed a joint Memorandum of Understanding on HIV/AIDS with the Jamaica Confederation of Trade Unions, Insurance and General Workers Trade Union in Trinidad and Tobago (BIGWU).

The above agreements are based on the following terms of references:

- Mobilizing partnership and building on existing structures
- Improving human resource capacity for effective delivery at country level.
- Facilitation by the UN System, Bridging work Place programmes and regional initiatives (Universal Access regional consultation.

Corporate Responses to HIV/AIDS-India Perspective

In January 2007, a study titled Corporate Responses to HIV/AIDS case studies by the World Bank and the Tata Research Institute suggested an early prevention of HIV/AIDS reduces the higher cost of treatment, death, disability and caring for people living with HIV and AIDS especially at the place of work. Sincere efforts by corporate houses can make effective and meaningful contribution in bringing awareness and prevention programmes concerning HIV and AIDS Epidemic at work place.

In India the following corporate houses have initiated work place programmes aimed at harm reduction concerning HIV/AIDS, Drug Abuse (I.V) and Alcohol abuse among industrial workers.

- *Reliance Industries Limited* has set up a medical center at Hazira, Gujarat for HIV/AIDS Epidemic—Prevention programmes. Their activities include awareness initiative, testing HIV infection, Counseling and Anti retroviral therapy (ART) concerning AIDS Epidemic.
- *Hindustan Lever Limited* **has initiated** HIV/AIDS Epidemic awareness through rural entrepreneurs by promoting and distributing condom for safe sex.
- *DCM Shriram* **Consolidated Limited** has organized programmes concerning HIV/AIDS Epidemic Awareness and prevention at its plants in Kota, Rajasthan.
- *Tata Energy Research Institute* has initiated numerous HIV and AIDS Awareness and Prevention programmes basing on local culture, education and communication material and ART (Anti Retroviral Therapy) promotion with HIV/AIDS Epidemic messages (Tapes, Street plays etc). These activities are conducted at various industrial sites (Jamshedpur Tata).
- *Delhi Metro Rail Corporation* **(DMRC),** a public sector company conducts HIV infection, awareness and its prevention activities among migrant workers. Activities includes education awareness about HIV infection and promotion of condom use.
- *Transport Corporation of India* **(TCI)** This corporation recognizes the importance of truck drivers, cleaners and the vulnerability of the truckers for HIV infection due to their mobility and nature of work. TCI has initiated and established the network of clinics serving long distance, truck drivers and their assistants by providing treatments for STI (Sexually Transmitted Infections) and counseling service for preventing HIV, promoting usage of condoms, ART therapy and Drugs Harm Reduction programmes.

AIDS Threatens Indian Prosperity

Tata Steel promotes awareness among employees about a disease that as yet has no cure but is preventable—Yale Global, 30 Nov. 2006). Parmita Mitra Tata Steel as the leading steel producer "seriously takes the HIV/AIDS Epidemic, gets periodic updates on the disease. The company is located in Jharkhand, a State with a high risk migrant labourers and truckers that makes them more vulnerable to the virus because of their mobile nature of job (long distance transport truck drivers and their assistants).

The alarming escalating rate of HIV infection among industrial workers is quite evident in the rest of India especially Chennai. The prevalence of AIDS among industrial workers in Shookagiri, RayakottaI and Jawalagiri is of a great concern as mentioned by Rural Inter Disciplinary Development Society (RIDDS), a non-governmental organization dealing with Prevention and Control Project (APAC).

If present HIV/AIDS trends continue, economists worry that there may be a slowdown in India's economy.

To summarize, in addition to educational seminars and workshops concerning Safe Sex (Use of Condom), Drugs Harm Reduction (injecting drug use) alcohol abuse and life style of industrial workers there is an urgent need of expansion of Anti Retro-viral Therapy (ART) treatment which at present is not adequate.

Prevention of HIV/AIDS:
A Tripartite Response (ILO Project)

The ILO (International Labour Organization) under its project "Prevention of HIV/AIDS in the world of work a tripartite response" documented the HIV/AIDS experiences of eight leading private and public sector enterprises health workers and its link to production is one of the main reasons why enterprises have chosen to respond to HIV/AIDS in India. The project has selected the states of, West Bengal, Madhya Pradesh and Jharkhand.

Mr. Madhur Bajaj, Vice Chairman, Bajaj Auto Limited, has aptly described about ILO Kit titled "Enterprises and HIV/AIDS in India" in the following paragraph.

"A healthy work force is the biggest asset for the company, a healthy work force would mean less of absenteeism that translates into better productivity". It is worth mentioning the contribution of ITF (International Transport Workers Federation) in bringing Awareness and Prevention of HIV/AIDS among transport workers (Truck Drivers, Assistants and Industrial Workers) which is quite praise worthy.

HIV/AIDS IN CHINA
HIV/AIDSWORKPLACE EDUCATION PROGRAM

China has launched AIDS Prevention work on the country's 200 million migrant workers vulnerable to HIV infection and AIDS Epidemic. This programme is a three year education campaign to provide awareness and prevention about HIV/AIDS among migrant workers and their families concerning discrimination and stigma, protecting the employment rights of the people in the work place. Beijing's Health Bureau indicates eighty percent of programmes are being co-sponsored by Chinese and American governments.

Experts from the Ministry of Health estimate there are about 650,000 people living with HIV/AIDS in China.

Business committed to fight HIV/AIDS in China
ILO/UNAIDS Workshop Kerry Center in Beijing (March 30, 2006)

More than 100 business houses, civil society and government representatives from China and abroad participated in this workshop discussing the role of business houses in dealing with HIV/AIDS in China.

It was pointed out that business has an important role to play in a number of social issues such as HIV and AIDS Epidemic. Business houses can influence their employees through education, insurance, safety and wellness programmes. These activities are synonymous with good and ethical business practices.

HIV/AIDS in Europe and Central Asia
(Dublin Declaration)

In February 2004 a conference titled "Breaking the Barriers Partnerships to fight HIV/AIDS in Europe and Central Asia" made the following major declaration in Dublin, Ireland.

Poverty, under development and illiteracy are among the principal contributory factors to the spread of HIV/AIDS.

- The European and Central Asian Region have almost 2.1 million people living with HIV/AIDS
- There is a rapid spread of HIV in South Eastern Europe and Central Asia.
- The Prevention of HIV infection can take place through the promotion of Safer and Responsible sexual behaviour and practices, including through condom use.
- The high risk people for HIV infection are drug injectors and their sexual partners, men having sex with men (MSM), Sex Workers, trafficking women, prisoners, ethnic minorities and migrant population.
- HIV/AIDS crisis needs strong basic health care system and services to ensure universal and equitable access to HIV/AIDS prevention. Cross border treatment and care, sub regional and technical collaboration and sharing of best practices for prevention of HIV transmission involving civil society and faith-based organizations, as well as people living with HIV/AIDS is in progress.

HIV/AIDS in Canada and USA

HIV/AIDS in work place holds particular importance in Canada and USA where universal access to treatment is more readily available than elsewhere although stigma, discrimination and ignorance may impair the protection of rights and proper access to care and treatment, unions have dealt with HIV within the broader framework of health and safety, disability and equality rights.

HIV/AIDS IN Malaysia

HIV/AIDS poses a serious challenge to Malaysia human development. By the end of 2006 approximately 75,000 Malaysians were reported having HIV infection. About 75% of HIV/AIDS cases in Malaysia are among major injecting drug users.

Based on the country's plan to expand "Drug Harm Reduction programmes to 25,000 injecting drug users, it is projected that either by 2009 or 2010, the country should see "positive results" and achieve the Millennium Development Goals (MDG) on HIV / AIDS.

HIV/AIDS in Nepal, Pakistan and Bangladesh

Nepal is facing increase in HIV prevalence. In Terai Nepal 70 percent of clients of sex workers are truckers. The percentage of truckers visiting regularly sex workers range from 25 to 80 percent IDUS (Injecting Drug Users) and MSM (Men having sex with men) these are high risk HIV groups in Nepal, Pakistan and Bangladesh.

With six million truck drivers in India and one million in Pakistan, the impact of HIV/AIDS on trucking industry has important social and economic implications on the transport industry.

In Bangladesh—240 AIDS cases were diagnosed and 109 died. It is estimated (2004) there are 7500' HIV cases 82.5% never used condoms with commercial sexual workers. According to UNAIDS, in Pakistan, it is estimated 70,000 to 80,000 are HIV positive or 0.1 percent of the adult population of Pakistan until September 2004, MSM, Unsafe Sexual Behavior are major risk factors for spreading HIV and AIDS.

HIV/AIDS Education Programmes for Transport Workers

Numerous studies around the World have indicated prevalence of HIV and STIs Sexually transmitted infection, among transport workers because of their nature of work (long distance truckers). They become victims of HIV infection, hepatitis B, virus, syphilis and Gonorrhea etc.

It is gratifying to point out that International Transport Worker's Federation (ITWF) is doing an excellent job by organizing and implementing HIV/AIDS education programmes for its members in various countries. They have provided the following alarming data concerning HIV/AIDS among transport workers.

- STI prevalence rate among transport workers is of great concern in many countries.
- HIV infection in West Africa especially among truck drivers varies 3% to 32%.
- 16% of the drivers in South India were HIV positive.
- Uganda railways staff (5600) have died due to AIDS

- 22% of seafarers (Unicef and UNAIDS) in Mekong Region South East Asia may be infected with HIV.

Possible Reasons for HIV infection among transport workers

- Mobility (long distance transport workers)
- Inadequate medical facilities (STI treatment)
- Lack of Awareness and Prevention about HIV/AIDS Epidemic
- Alcohol and drug abuse especially injectible drug (IV drugs)
- Sexual harassment and deprivation due to inadequate resting, recreation and long distance traveling
- Frequent absence from home
- Work Load Stress and lack of peace of mind
- Indifferent community and law enforcement officials
- Harassment (police, border crossing officials).

Impact of HIV/AIDS on Workers

- Fear, Stigma and discrimination
- Absentism from work
- Loss of income
- Fear of Inadequate screening/testing (HIV virus) Unsure of confidential reporting
- Fear of dismissal or losing job due to HIV infection
- Loss of employee benefits
- Not effective support from Unions

Salient Features of HIV/AIDS Education Programmes for Industrial Workers

The following are some suggested salient features which may be considered in the education programmes concerning HIV and AIDS Epidemic for workers:

- Adequate knowledge about HIV and AIDS and its prevention
- Promoting Healthy life style (Values clarification and behaviour change)
- Blending of Modern and Traditional Values among young industrial workers

- Voluntary counseling, testing of HIV infection with confidentiality.
- The role of ART in HIV/AIDS prevention.

Anti Retroviral Treatment (ART) and Prevention of HIV/AIDS through Education

i.   HIV/ AIDS is not curable but it can be treated
ii.   ART prolongs lives—AIDS a chronic disease not a death sentence
iii. ART may calm fears and change attitude towards life
iv.   ART, integrated with prevention can reduce HIV transmission
v.   ART, no doubt very expensive but is now much more affordable.
vi.   ART can return sick people back to productive lives.
vii. Overcoming stigma and discrimination of HIV infection.
viii. Mobile clinics and trained para medicos in rural areas to visit workers HIV positive families for prevention for AIDS through education.

Ref: Avoiding HIV infection in the Work place

(Ref www.dshs.state.tx.us/hivstd)

The following good personal hygienic practices may be practiced in the work place as most people could be exposed to HIV if they had another round.

i.   Keep broken skin covered with a clean, dry bandage
ii.   Avoid direct contact with blood spills
iii. Wear gloves to clean spills that contain visible blood; and
iv.   Clean blood spills with an appropriate disinfectant or 1:10 solution of freshly mixed household bleach and water. After cleaning, wash hands thoroughly with soap and running water.

According to Dr. Peter Piot of UNAID "In order to prevent the spread of HIV, a combination approach is required. We need to promote abstinence, delay of sex, faithfulness and the use of condoms. No single approach will work and for any program to be effective, information, education, drug harm reduction (IDUs) and support counseling materials are essential. This can be achieved only by establishing a clinic or training center for bringing about HIV/AIDS Awareness and its Prevention."

To sum up, we quote Dr. Piot, UNAIDS Executive Director

"Until we recognize AIDS as the development and security issue of our time, we cannot succeed in beating the Epidemic."

The author in this Hand Book has discussed the following topics in the proceeding chapters with special reference to India in the light of Introduction chapter.

- Present scenario of HIV/AIDS among Industrial workers with reference to Transport workers.
- Life style and Attitudes of young Industrial workers
- Healthy living
- HIV/AIDS and its prevention
- Cultural Heritage and Sexual Behavior Pattern in India and Third World countries
- Clarification of Values and HIV/AIDS Prevention.
- Psychic Drugs (Intravenous), HIV/AIDS and Alcohol abuse among industrial workers.
- Role of Management, Unions and Community Awareness Drive in Preventing HIV/AIDS through education.

REFERENCES

- Poverty and HIV /AIDS in Africa, 2002, Third World Quarterly, Vol. 23, No.2, PP 313332 http/www.
- HIV, AIDS and the work place, 2006, Texas Department of State Health Service HIV/STD comprehensive services Branch www.
- ILO/AIDS and the World of work in Latin America and the Caribbean: May 2006 opportunities and challenges.
- CHINA.ORG.CN China Launches HIV/AIDS work place Education Program
- Business committed to fight. HIV/AIDS in China, March 30, 2006 Press Release, United Nations Development Program.
- HIV/AIDS: Transport workers take action. International Transport Workers Federation (ITF),
- HIV /AIDS and Transport: Time for global response. International Transport Workers Federation.
- Corporate Responses to HIV/AIDS in India 2003. The World Bank
- S. Parsad, Prevalence of AIDS among Industrial Workers, Dec. 2007 The Hindu, India's National Newspaper
- AIDS Threatens Indian Prosperity, Yale Global on line.

CHAPTER 1

Present Scenario of AIDS among Industrial Workers

Life is no brief candle to me. It is a sort of splendid torch which I have got hold of for the moment and I want to make it burn as brightly as possible before handing it on to future generations.

George Bernard Shaw

The monster AIDS (Acquired Immuno Deficiency Syndrome) is attacking our industrial workers. AIDS knows no boundaries and does not discriminate against anyone. It kills and there is no known cure or vaccine for it. It is mainly contracted through sexual activity like other sexually transmitted diseases and also through blood transfusion and intravenous drug use.

AIDS is strikingly common among the weaker sections i.e., factory workers and daily-wage earners. In the industrial township of Faridabad, as many as 18 cases of HIV positive and AIDS were registered in the last 15 months—seven in the Escorts Medical Centre and 1 in the B.K. Hospital (Faridabad).

A couple of years ago, we were caught napping with no strategy planned on how to deal with emergencies like Plague. We should not be placed in a similar situation in coping with the menace of AIDS, which is expected to hit India the hardest in the coming years. According to Experts, India in 5 years time may well overtake Africa as the epicenter of AIDS.

HIV and AIDS among Truck Drivers in J & K (Transport Industry)

Jammu and Kashmir is one of the most important states, due to domestic and international tourism. Transport industry is one of the major links with other Sates like Delhi, Maharashtra, Tamil Nadu, West Bengal, Punjab and Haryana, for transporting fruits like apples, cherries, almonds and walnuts etc., from J&K, Approximately fifteen thousand trucks employing four thousand personnel are plying in the state. These truckers are frequently away from their families for a considerable time (sometimes may be weeks or months together). Hence the temptation to indulge in sexual affairs (may be with commercial sex workers) and using narcotic drugs at places of their halt and rest on national highways is always there. Thus, they are potential HIV patients and also high risk HIV carriers. Generally they are from rural background and are likely to spread the disease to their family members. A study titled HIV Surveillance and AIDS Education of Truckers in J&K was conducted by Dr. Rajender Singh sponsored by Department of Science and Technology, Government of J&K, India. The sample for this study were one thousand truckers randomly selected.

Major Findings of the Study

1. Transport industry (truckers) form one of the most important potential high risk group for HIV / AIDS.
2. Most of the truckers (52%) were in the age group of 16-25 years.
3. The literacy of the truckers was poor (28% were totally illiterate and 49% had primary education).
4. 78% of truckers had been indulging in extra-marital sexual relations (74-6%—hetrosexual and 2% homosexual).
5. 80.8%were not using condoms.
6. Drug addiction (75%), cigarette smoking (71 %), Chutki and Pan Masala (62%) were the major addictions.
7. Awareness regarding HIV/AIDS was almost negligible. Most of the truckers were not knowledgeable about modes of transmission (blood transfusion, narcotic drug abuses and multiple sex partners) and prevention of AIDS.

RecommendationS of the study

➤ Audio-cassettes in different languages should be distributed to the truckers for educating them regarding prevention of AIDS
➤ Video-Cassettes and street plays should be organized on highways or places of trucker's rest.
➤ Banners, posters and hoardings regarding prevention of AIDS at the transport offices where driving licences are issued.
➤ Frequent surveillance of truckers should be carried out regarding importance of AIDS education in their lifestyle and attitudes.

As the lifestyle of industrial workers is similarly risky the above study provides a scenario of potential spread of HIV Epidemic among industrial workers as well because most of the labour force consists of migrant workers.

To have an in-depth analysis of the above situation, one may have to deliberate upon the changing values, outlooks and lifestyles of these industrial workers in the context of contemporary scenario of industrial growth.

KAB Study on AIDS Awareness among Hotel Employees (Madras, 1993)

This study was conducted by Dr. Usha and Sayee Kumar in Chennai involving different levels of hotels. 40 questions regarding AIDS awareness were administered to 1000 hotel employees. 79 persons were aware of condoms, only 55 agreed that condoms can prevent AIDS. 23 persons had admitted to having multipartnered sex.

It is worth mentioning here that inspite of high level of awareness; many hotel employees are still having multipartnered sex without condom.

Condom Promotion and Education of Sex Workers through Sex Brokers and Clients in Madras, India.

This study was conducted in Kodambula, Vadapalami and K.K. Nagar to intervene in the prostitution areas of Chennai with AIDS awareness and prevention programmes. This project involves not only the sex workers but clients, brothel aunties, brothel runners, the sex surrounding industry etc. IEC base line was conducted to assess condom usage rates, which at present is below 10%.

Industrial Growth and Lifestyle, Attitudes of Industrial Workers in India—Present Scenario

As the scenario of industrial growth and development has been rapidly changing due to liberalization and modernization in the industrial sector and collaboration with multinationals, life styles, attitudes, values and outlooks of industrial workers are undergoing drastic changes, the age old customs have lost their relevance and adoption of pseudo-western values has become the fashion of the day. Exposure through the multimedia communication system has brought sexual permissiveness among youth.

Young industrial workers generally belong to low socio-economic section of society and are compelled by poverty to leave their schools and homes in rural areas to work in big industrial towns and cities. Being young and frustrate they indulge in sex, which puts them at great risk of contracting sexually transmitted diseases. They are also unconcerned to find out on their own any information about prevention of AIDS through safety measures. Generally, they are ignorant about health risks due to their actions. Since these industrial workers move from one job to another, from one place to another, their mobility puts them at greater risk of contracting sexually transmitted disease and consequently HIV / AIDS infection. Further these workers are forced to live in slums or chawls or in cramped rooms (due to poverty) and sleep in close contact with other workers. Therefore, their sexual behaviour could involve homosexuality, bisexuality or just any other unhealthy sex habit. Thus the above scenario has ramification on lifestyles and attitudes of the industrial workers which has been discussed in detail in the next chapters.

Suggested line of action for Truck Drivers & HIV / AIDS Epidemic

Due to the nature of truck drivers' work that involves long hours of driving on highways full of risks and general difficulties, life for them is an uncertain journey, full of stress and strain. As these truck drivers leave their families away sometimes in remote rural areas and have practically no real home to stay at night for a long duration, they are quite lonesome and frustrated.

The monotony and the anxiety causes boredom and tensions. For several reasons the truck drivers tend to ignore the risk of drinking while driving. The prevalence of alcoholism drug abuse and unsafe sex is high among truck drivers.

Thus having unsafe sex at unknown unhygienic places with an affordable sex worker makes them vulnerable to all kinds of sexually transmitted infections (STI). They are at a greater risk of exposure to HIV/AIDS as well. Because of their wandering lifestyle they can be the most risky agents for spreading the disease—passing on the infection to their wives and multiple partners. The following are some suggestions for HIV/AIDS Awareness and Prevention among truck drivers.

Practical Strategies to prevent HIV/AIDS Epidemic among Truck Drivers

EDUCATION

➢ Awareness about nature of HIV / AIDS
➢ Frequent and constant reminders about HIV/AIDS Prevention
➢ Consequences and impact of HIV / AIDS on family (Wife and Children).
➢ Stigma and Discrimination of HIV infection in the community and society.

II SAFE STOP STATION

➢ Safe halt stations on the main highway
➢ Bed / lodging / Food available on road side motels/Dhabas
➢ Licenced Sex Workers to have regular medical check-up.
➢ Availability of quality condoms.

III HIV /AIDS KNOWLEDGE

➢ Bill boards and signs on the highways
➢ Messages on the truck tail boards—Avoid HIV/AIDS
➢ Hand outs concerning HIV/AIDS Awareness and its Prevention in different languages (local and regional languages)

IV NGO's (Non Government Organization)

➢ Sponsorships to genuine NGOs
➢ Involving spiritual leaders conveying HIV/AIDS Prevention in their discourses, camps and seminars. (Temple/Mosque/Church) with emphasis on love and loyality towards family.
➢ Tax shelters to NGOs working on HIV/AIDS issues.

Management Responsibility

➢ HIV/AIDS Awareness and Prevention workshops / seminars
➢ Medical Check-up at recruitment which may include HIV testing.
➢ Frequent (annual) comprehensive medical check-up
➢ Voluntary HIV testing with assurance of confidentiality
➢ Medical insurance for the family
➢ Where possible provide affordable housing enroute or affordable company owned and well managed shelters for rest breaks.

VI. GOVERNMENT responsibility

➢ Awareness and prevention of the HIV/AIDS Epidemic trough education at all levels.
➢ Driver's training schools to include HIV/AIDS prevention/ education to students
➢ Proper surveillance of highway halts and provision of government rest homes.
➢ Incentives to corporate houses for providing a healthy environment for employees.
➢ Subsidized health care for industrial and transport workers.

CHAPTER 2

Lifestyle and Attitudes of Young Industrial Workers

Recently there has been widespread interest in understanding the youth, particularly the young industrial worker. As the scenario of industrial growth and development has been rapidly changing due to strides in science and technology, lifestyles, attitudes, values and outlooks of industrial workers are rapidly changing. This is indeed a relatively new field of research and is attracting considerable attention from sociologists, psychologists, educationists and political leaders. While this field of research is of relevance to developed countries, it has paramount importance to developing countries, since they are going through a sensitive phase of transformation from poverty to comfortable life for their vast, ever growing population.

Contributing Factors Relating to the Lifestyles of Industrial Workers

The following are some major contributing factors for their life styles and attitudes of industrial workers especially young workers.

(A) The Family: Blood Relations: In India the role of family is very important as a socializing institution for young industrial workers. This is primarily due to traditional, cultural and religious bonds, which exist between individuals and family members. Although the situation is now rapidly changing in cities, particularly amongst literate segments of the population, among the industrial workers the role of family has not lost its importance. However, it should be noted that joint family structure is cracking and so the extent of influence of the family is also diminishing.

The role of old parents continues to be important in running the family matters because of the Indian patriarchal society structure particularly in rural areas. Nevertheless, the rigid dogmatic values founded on religious and traditional belief are increasingly less acceptable to the young generation. This has resulted into a greater degree of tension prevailing in the family. Despite this in a majority of working class families the situation is authoritarian, i.e. the father controlling the affairs. Considering the background of joint family structure, in order to avoid confrontation and minimize tension, young industrial workers try to get as far away as possible from their homes, especially in cities. If the worker is still in a joint family, his involvement with family affairs still continues to dominate his non-working hours.

(B) Other types of family and sex: In view of a very high degree of religious values prevailing in the Indian society, sex is considered a subject of high moral value. Despite the changing scene of Indian society, pre-marital sex or homosexuality is not only unacceptable, but is considered to be a moral or a social evil. All the same, the rigid barriers of caste, creed, religion, region are crumbling slowly and inter-caste marriages, and selection of a spouse of their own choice is increasingly gaining momentum.

In India, the importance of sex education is not considered either by parents or by educational governmental authorities. This is primarily due to, high moral values and religious taboos attached to sex. This lack of knowledge of sex among young industrial workers compiled with lack of sufficient leisure or recreational facilities, leads to a lot of mental tensions and frustrations, which psychologically affect the work output as well as personal life of an individual. The fall out of this appears to manifest itself in having more children, which confounds to the vicious cycle of poverty and family tension. This compels the women folk to seek employment to augment the family income. A major drive started by the Government of India on the family planning education has started yielding some results primarily in urban areas.

(C) Education: The major industrial workforce in India can be classified in two categories—semi-literate and illiterate. It is only in modern industries such as Pharmaceutical, Chemical Fertilizers and Electronics etc., where the workforce is literate. This is mainly due to the growing population and lack of sufficient resource on the part of government to provide minimum education. The financial problem of working class families does not allow them to educate their children. Putting them to work at an early age to generate extra income to make both ends meet seems to be the only way of survival.

In rural India, family and neighborhood environment by and large have remained unaffected by the cultural revolution. Existence of religious and ethnic traditions are depriving youngsters, particularly girls, of formal education. As a matter of fact the ignorance and rigid attitude of old people is blocking the young generations' education. Realizing the problems, the Government of India in 1950 launched non-formal education and adult education programmes on a massive scale in rural India.

The increasing awareness of educational need in many working families is giving rise to new problems—on one hand there is a generation gap and on the other hand there is a huge social gap between young workers with some schooling background and those with none. The former prefer to seek employment in urban towns and attempt to lead a more civilized life. There resisting the idea of returning to their native place which could be a backward rural area. Consequently the literate young people from rural India do not contribute much to the cultural and social revolution of rural India.

One major point which has come to surface of late is the need of job-oriented education visa-vis the standard curriculum used by educational authorities. Most of the subjects that are taught in schools are found to be of very little significance at the work place. The method and contents of educational curriculum vis-a-vis the economic and social needs of India are found to be perpendicular to each other. It is with this discovery that now the Government has started moving in the direction where job-oriented education would be given more emphasis.

Yet another problem faced by India is, a large work-force trained for specific responsibilities which remain unemployed and are forced by circumstances to accept jobs at a level below their professional capacities. This leads to:

  i.   Frustration
  ii. Low productivity
  iii. Industrial unrest
  iv. Migration to other developed countries

It would not be out of place to mention here that India possesses the third largest technical workforce in the world and has been losing a substantial work-force to the developed/industrialized/ rich nations of the world.

Many parents, having realized that normal school education would not provide a desired background for their children for the work life, have started utilizing the technical institutions increasingly. Industrial Training Institutes' (ITI) programmes are gaining popularity.

(D) Work: Unemployment is the second major problem of India. In the urban areas with the changing life style of society at large, young members of working class families seek a decent employment. Due to scarcity of jobs they remain unemployed for a longer period without contributing any income to the family pool. As such today it is the young who are hardest hit by unemployment.

With a lot of young males seeking jobs, the opportunities for young women are minimized. In India one sees that women workforce is employed for a typical kind of operation, which is best suited for women. In most of the cases women workforce is not considered at par with the males.

Most of the young men of working class families find themselves at a loss after completion of education because they are not in a position to plan their future. The unemployment and poverty is accepted as part of one's life which tends to result in developing negative and rigid attitudes towards society.

With the availability of huge work force in India, social welfare and additional facilities are not provided by the employers which also results in industrial accidents besides affecting the health of the workers. In many cases it is also found that the family type of organizations exploit the labor market by depriving right compensation to the workforce viz., temporary employments, low job security benefits such as provident fund, gratuity and medical facilities.

Young working people in India have another hazard of discrimination due to their age. They are paid less for the same job than adults.

There is another category of young job seekers who migrate from rural areas to big cities where they find that getting a meaningful employment is not very easy. In most of the cities this class of young workers creates a unique kind of problem. Many of the cities of India are plagued by the problems created by the influx of migratory workers and have come to a stage of breakdown. Places like Kolkata, Kanpur, are glaring examples. The first symptoms of these frustrated young people are violence, industrial unrest, unlawful activities, crimes etc.

The Government of India's policy of dispersal of industries away from the urban centers which was adopted in the Five Year Plans has started paying dividends thereby minimizing the exodus of rural young people to cities.

(E) Leisure & Culture: leisure is really an extracurricular activity for young people in India. It is the means to seek pleasure as an antidote to the work and family tensions. Considering the resources available for spending on leisure activities, the young industrial workers in India tend to involve in the following activities: native games, native cultural events such as Durga Puja in West Bengal, Ganesh Festival in Maharashtra, Mattu Pongal in Tamil Nadu, Navratri in Gujarat, Baisakhi in Punjab etc. Traditional fairs, melas, Onams, carnivals, also attract substantial number of young people especially in rural India. The Indian scene is dominated by a mix of cultural events as well as purely entertainment-oriented activities. Whereas the values attached to the cultural events by the old timers are more sentimental, the younger generation participate in these activities for fun only Cinema going habit is the most favourite amongst the young working class.

The concept of community centers as a place for recreation has been gaining momentum since 1960. The community centers as such can be attributed to an initiative from the Government, which was later followed, by the employers and philanthropists. The widespread TV network proposed in the current five year plan is expected to provide another important source of leisure for a large section of young working class people. Folk music, dance, plays etc. have also contributed to the social life of many young people in India. Most of these activities are very much in line with the local cultural and traditional background.

Most of the young industrial workers in India by and large consider physical fitness very important. As such they are found to be engaged in activities like exercise or sports or games, which contribute to physical fitness.

Considering the fact that the government, semi-government or social bodies' efforts to provide leisure have their own limitations, primarily because of the constricted resources of local clubs in which the organizers have been making attempts to organize such activities. However, the efforts are far from satisfactory. A government organization set up to look after the youth welfare in the Third, Five Year Plan under the banner 'Nehru Yuvak Kendras' has been quite successful in this direction, though in a limited way.

(F) Participation & Alienation: In India the organized Trade Union movement has been gathering momentum for the last two decades. It is unfortunate that some Trade Union movement instead of improving the working conditions of workers and productivity has been resulting into confrontation, thereby working against the interests of workers. This is normally triggered off and exploited by the vested interest parties or by political institutions. Young industrial workers who are emotional and frustrated fall into this trap, thereby disturbing the harmony of the industry and workers. The Indian workers mostly get involved into the radical movements organized for a specific cause rather than joining a permanent movement created for achievement of some ideological objectives. However, considering the magnitude of unemployment and disparity of income among various classes of population the vested interests tend to vitiate these activities for their personal gains. While a majority of the industrial workers in urban India involve themselves in organized movements the scene is different in rural India. Because of the strong cultural bonds and prevailing illiteracy, these young people eliminate themselves from major organized movements. This scene is much different from the pre-independence era when the nationalists ideals and sentiments used to make the rural youngster follow the organized movements of freedom struggle.

The widespread acceptance of industrial democracy as the institutional metric for resolution of conflicts between the employers and employees and the emulation of participative management have resulted in a new awakening and consciousness in the educated and organized segment of Indian industrial workers. Not content with the established means of asserting themselves they are seeking new ways of venting their grievances for redressal including manifestation of militancy and violence.

To summarize as a consequence of the changing lifestyle and changing values, unfulfilled aspirations unceration future, economic and social disparities, unemployment and employment that enforces young workers to snap ties with their families and move from rural to urban areas where the young industrial workers live in crowded shelters with their meager income—all these factors when combined together make the young vulnerable to all kinds of diseases. Their sexual life under these circumstances is far from what it should be. Indicators point out inherent danger of AIDS monster attacking these workers. Thus, it is imperative that industrialists, social scientists, the media and the government join hands in preventing the AIDS time bomb explosion, among young industrial workers who are the backbone of our economy. As we are already aware that there is no vaccine for AIDS prevention, the only way of prevention is through Education and bringing awareness regarding preventing AIDS strategies among industrial workers in India.

CHAPTER 3

Cultural Heritage and Sexual Behaviour Pattern in India

As we are aware of the fact that HIV/AIDS is a Sexually Transmitted infection, it is imperative to have insight about the sexual behavior patterns and traditions prevailing in India.

According to the Upanishads, the philosophical version of the earlier Vedas (Hindu scriptures), Manu ji has divided life into four stages or orders:

1. Brahmacharya, or the period of student life.
2. Grihesth, or married life
3. Vanaprastha, or the period of ascetic life devoted to the perfection of character, the study of spiritual science and divine contemplation.
4. Sanyas, or the period of renunciation devoted to the preaching of truth and righteousness all over the world by abandoning all worldly connections.

The first stage i.e., Brahamcharya encompasses the adolescent stage. The following five characteristics are indicated: (i) Always speak the truth, (ii) Lead a virtuous life; (iii) Abstain from sexual indulgence; (iv) Never be negligent in learning and teaching (v) Devote yourself to sciences (physical and spiritual) till your knowledge is perfect.

To summarise, a Brahmachari (student) should abstain from the following five kinds of sexual excitement in relation to persons of the opposite sex.

i.   Looking upon them with an eye of lust;
ii.   Embracing them;
iii. Having sexual intercourse with them;
iv.   Reading or talking of libidinous subjects;
v.   Indulging in lascivious thoughts i.e. mental intercourse with persons of opposite sex.

Upanishads and Sexual Abstinence

Thus, abstinence from sex was considered a virtue in the ancient scriptures of Indian heritage. One could "realize the self" by practicing asceticism (tapas) which include abstinence from sex as an essential element.

Through the observance of 'brahmacharya'—the total abstinence from sex in thought, word and deed—semen could be converted into ojas and moved upwards to the brain. In that case, it became a source of physical and spiritual strength.

Mahatma Gandhi and Sexual Abstinence

Mahatama Gandhi was a strong advocate of total sexual abstinence except for furthering generation. His following statement reiterates the traditional notion about loss of energy through loss of semen (Gandhi, 1943:71):

Once the idea that the only and grand function of the sexual organ is generation, possesses men and women, union for any other purpose they will hold as criminal waste of precious energy. It is now easy to understand why the scientists of old have put such great value upon the vital fluid and why they have insisted upon its strong transmutation into the highest form of energy for the benefit of society.

Sex Sublimating to Spirituality

The traditional aspiration of sublimating sexuality into spirituality through abstinence in Hindu culture had made a strong impact on thoughts and actions of people in ancient India. Only a fraction of contemporary

Hindus may have practiced total abstinence from sex for spiritual gain, but the theory of sublimation was widely known (Kakkar, 1989). In a simple and layman's version, the theory states that virya—which stands for both vigour and semen—is the fountain of physical as well as spiritual strength and that the loss of virya through sexual act or imagery is not conducive for health from physical and spiritual point of view. Some believe that virya can either move downwards in sexual intercourse and emitted in its gross physical form as semen or it can move upwards through spinal cord to the brain in a form known as 'ojas'.

Some Common Beliefs regarding Virya (Semen)

According to ancient scriptures in India, food is converted into semen by successive transformations through blood, flesh, fat, bone and marrow (Kakkar, 1989). A few common assumptions are: (i) 40 drops of blood produce one drop of semen; (ii) each ejaculation involves a loss of half an ounce of semen, which requires consumption of 60 pounds of food; and (iii) each copulation is equivalent to energy expenditure by 24 hours of concentrated mental activity or 72 hours of hard physical labor.

Modern Culture and Sexual Abstinence

The modern trend in India is to criticize the idea of preaching sexual abstinence to unmarried boys and girls. The dominant view is that it is useless to stress sexual abstinence in sex education curricula of schools because it will simply turn off the students, who are exposed to sex and violence through T.V media and a large proportion of whom may have already been engaged in sexual relations. It is also suggested that condoms become more easily available to them by making them available in schools. But, the author still believes that in the present context with special reference to rapid spread of HIV/STD infection, it may be necessary to emphasise abstinence from premarital and multiple sexual relationship. This is also in accordance to our cultural heritage and is a viable option for protection from HIV infection.

Other Sexual Behaviour Patterns in India

(A) Prostitution: Prostitution or the practice of indulging in promiscuous sexual relations for money or other favours is an ancient institution in India. Kautilya's Artha in circa 300 B.C., has aptly described female sex workers regarding the norms, behaviour, prerogatives and responsibilities (Basham, 1959: 184).

(B) Devadasi: Devadasi system of purchasing young girls and dedicating them to temples, which often made them objects of sexual pleasure for temple priests and others, was an age-old custom in some parts of India, especially in southern India. By 300 A.D gods in some Hindu temples were treated like kings; tlley had wives, but had also unmarried women known as devadasis (handmaidens of God), who attended to gods' persons, danced and sang before them, and bestowed sexual favours on the courtiers whom he favoured. Male worshippers gave generous funds to the temple. These women called devadasis were often the offsprings of mothers of the same profession, born and reared in the temple compounds.

But devadasis often became victims of sexual exploitation by temple priests as well as pilgrims and now have been compelled to take to prostitution either on a regular or part-time basis.

(C) Homosexuality: Another sexual behaviour pattern which was recognized in ancient India (Vatsayanan's Kama Sutra refers to it) was the practice of oral sex by eunuchs with their male patrons and by male servants with their masters. (Burton and Arbutnnot, 93:62-65), Lesbian acts are depicted in the erotic sculptures of medieval Hindu temples (Lal, 966:plates 67 and 68).

During the Muslim rule in India, homosexuality entered Indian court life. Some Muslim rulers are reported to have maintained harems of young boys.

The word in vogue in the western hemisphere regarding homosexual is "gay". Both male homosexuals and female homosexuals (lesbians) are classified as "gays". In modern times, it usually refers to persons whose predominant erotic inclination is towards their own sex whether or not they engage themselves in homosexual behaviour.

(D) Hijras: The commonly used English translation of the Urdu word "Hijra" is 'eunuch'. A less commonly used translation is 'intersex (hermaphrodite). 'Eunuch' refers to a castrated (emasculated) male and 'intersex' refers to a person whose genitals are ambiguously male-like at birth. Impotence is the force behind both the English words but is only a necessary and not a sufficient condition for being recognized as hijra in India.

Hijras are popular in the northern part of India where they carry on their traditional roles of dancing and singing in homes on occasions of male childbirth, wedding and other festivals.

Anthropologists believe that in addition to their traditional cultural role as performers for means of livelihood, they also engage in sexual activity with men for money or for satisfying their own sexual desires.

Strategies for Safe Sex

As pointed out earlier, the concept about the value of sexual abstinence among young industrial workers in modern India is not very practical. Even from Catholic point of view "to sacrifice sex privileges by a celibate life is superior to the use of generative function if it is undertaken for the purpose of freeing oneself for an even nobler service of God" (Ciemens, 1961:236). Many psychologists consider prolonged abstinence detrimental to marital and physical health.

However, it is worth mentioning that people should be discouraged from premarital sex with reference to their cultural heritage. If it is not feasible in the modern environment, it may be desirable to discuss safe strategies for sex so that they do not get infected with AIDS/HIV infection. Thus to protect oneself especially at the adolescent stage from STD (Sexually Transmitted Diseases), strategies for safe sex need to be deliberated upon.

Use of Condom

The statistics regarding number of condom users increased from 3 per cent in 1970 to only 5 per cent in 1988-89, while the total contraceptive prevalence increased from 14 per cent in 1970 to 43 per cent in 1988-93. For reasons not yet understood, Indian States/Union Territories vary considerably in their choice of condom as a contraceptive method.

It protects couples both from unwanted pregnancy and sexually transmitted infection like AIDS/HIV infection. The main constraints on the use of condoms in India are:

i.   Lack of good quality
ii.   Less effectiveness
iii.   Inadequate knowledge and advantages of use of Condoms
iv.   Cultural Sensitivity
v.   Storage and disposal problems
vi.   Reduced pleasure of sexual intercourse
vii.   Interruption in the sex act by the use of condom, thereby reducing the pleasure, and
viii. Thickness of the condom making the use even painful in absence of lubricating gels.

With the hovering danger of the AIDS pandemic, mainly through unprotected sexual intercourse, an intervention program for much wider use of condoms than at present, particularly among groups vulnerable to this killer disease, AIDS should be a matter of top most priority.

Sexually Exploited Groups—Young Industrial Workers

Other sexually exploited groups are out-of-school adolescents. This may include young industrial workers. These groups are highly vulnerable to HIV/STD infection and perhaps have even less control over their sexual relations than Female Sex Workers which include adolescent boys and girls employed in organized and non-organized sectors who become victims of rape and sodomy. Homeless (often orphan) boys and girls who live a hand-to-mouth existence by working in Dhabas, on railway platforms, as rag pickers and in whatever odd jobs (Truck drivers, cleaners & helpers) available to them during the daytime, and sleep under bridges, parks and railway stations in cities, are easy victims of sexual exploitations by many men including those who have some control over these public places. The exploiters are likely to belong to high risk groups regarding HIV/STD infection. Thus, it is imperative to orient these sexually exploitated groups especially young industrial workers about the safe sex practices.

CHAPTER 4

AIDS & Its Prevention

To discuss pointers on AIDS, it is imperative to have basic and fundamental knowledge about AIDS/HIV infection in a very simple manner.

I.   *Introduction*

— HIV infection is a killer disease since there is no vaccine and no cure.
— It is mainly a sexually transmitted disease (STD)
— It was identified in 1984 by French and American scientists but the human immune deficiency virus did not get its name until 1986.
— According to newspapers and reports by various health organization—"AIDS will kill 10,000 Indians a day by the end of this century.
— It is estimated that 5,000 women will be widowed and 20,000 children will be orphaned daily in the country.

The scenario in other third world countries is very pessimistic. The killer disease is spreading like wild fire. But we can prevent this killer disease through adequate care, guidance and due precautions. Let us first discuss about the genesis of AIDS.

II.   *AIDS—what is it?*

1) The body health is defended by its immune system. White blood cells called, Lymphocytes i.e. B& T cells protect the body from germs (such as viruses, bacteria, parasites and fungi)

2) When germs are detected in the body system, B & T cells are activated and produce antibody to combat the invading foreign bodies.

3) This process is hindered in case of Acquired Immuno Deficiency Syndrome (AIDS)

   AIDS is a disease in which the body's immune system breaks down. AIDS is caused by the Human Immuno Deficiency Virus (HIV)

4) When HIV enters the body it infects special T cells. "The virus kills these cells slowly. As more and more of the T Cells die, the body's ability to fight infection weakens.

Modes of HIV/AIDS spread in India

Heterosexual	72%
Blood Transfusion	12%
Intravenous Drug User	4%
Spouses of AIDS Patients	4%
Blood Products	3%
Homosexual	1%
Others	6%

V.   *HIV Infection and Illness*

HIV infection can lead to AIDS after a few years.

AIDS diagnoses—People suffering from fully developed AIDS symptoms for a breakdown of the immune system can be diagonozed with special tests for detecting the presence of antibodies, window period for HIV infection varies from 2 to 10 years.

A. *What are the symptoms?*

(i) Unexpected weight loss

(ii) Enlarged glands

(iii) Night sweats

(iv) Swollen lump glands in the neck, armpit or groin

(v) Diarrhoea, fevers, chills

(vi) Dry coughs

(vii) In some cases, a severe temporary illness.

It must be pointed out that a person infected with HIV may live on symptom free for 6 months to 2 years. Therefore awareness about the HIV status of your partners is absolutely essential before any sexual relationships. Ignorance about the infections leads to rapid spread of HIV if the infected person has sex with multiple partners without any precaution.

(b) *Modes of HIV transmission*

1. **Heterosexual activity** without precautions. Intercourse without precautions (use of condoms) may cause AIDS.
2. **Blood transfusion** People suffering from haemophilia or undergoing any major surgery: must ensure screening of blood before transfusion. It is mandatory to test the donors blood for HIV.
3. **Intravenously** Drug users sharing a needle or syringe containing blood from an infected person.
4. Hiv positive women can transmit the virus to **new born babies or even to the foetus in their womb.**

To sum up, any activity which includes the transfer of saliva sputum with infected blood, semen or vaginal fluids from an infected person into the blood stream of another person can be a source of HIV infection.

(c) *Who can get it?*

(a) Heterosexual without safe sex
(b) Drug users (IV)
(c) Homosexuals
(d) New—born babies from infected mothers.
(e) Foetus in infected mother's womb.

VI.   *Some MYTHS about getting HIV Infection / AIDS*

You cannot get AIDS:

(i)   By kissing, touching or hugging someone or by sharing eatables.
(ii) By drinking water from fountains.
(iii) By sharing articles of daily use such as telephones, utensils, papers, toilet seats, towels or through a person having a cough or bad cold.
(iv) By donating blood (if disposable or sterilized needles are used.

(v) From daily routine activity such as going to religious places, schools or grocers.

VII. *A Few suggestions for Prevention of AIDS*

(a) Avoid pre-marital extra / marital casual sexual relationships Sex with one known partner is safer.

(b) Respect for sex: clean, positive and healthy relationship.

(c) If sexual relationship is totally unavoidable, use condoms to prevent exchange of body fluids from start to finish.

(d) Avoid mixing with multiple partners

(e) Do not use drugs, especially intravenously (infected and unsterilized needles may cause AIDS)

(f) Before blood transfusion, one may make sure for uninfected blood (free from HIV infection).

(g) Though kissing and hugging does not cause infection—intimate kissing when gums or teeth ate infected can result in getting the infection through infected blood or saliva of the person who is HIV positive.

CHAPTER 5

Psychic Drugs, AIDS, Alcohol and Industrial Workers

(A curriculum unit for the counselors of the non-formal center)

They might not need me, but they might
I'll let my head be just in sight
A smile as small as mine might be
Precisely their necessity

Emily Dickinson

This chapter deals with major categories of drugs. Medicinal uses and abuses of miscellaneous tranquillizers, narcotics, hallucinogens, stimulants, sedatives. Suggested activities regarding awareness of drug pushing, production, etc. and its relationship with AIDS/HIV infection & abuses of Alcohol have been discussed.

The main objectives being-

(i)   To understand the meaning of a drug,
(ii) To provide comprehensive knowledge on the effects of abuse, so that industrial workers especially young ones may know the harmful effects of IV (intravenous) drugs and its relationship with AIDS/HIV infection.
(iii) to familiarize industrial workers with various psychic drugs, used by addicts and pushers.

Note: This is an informative unit on drugs. lecturing alone may not motivate the workers. It may be desirable to impart comprehensive knowledge about drugs among industrial workers in an interesting manner, either through discussions or screening of films and lectures by experts. Since the literacy level of some of the young industrial workers may not be very good, more stress should be laid on verbal participation and discussions in the counseling center.

Contents	Examples, Apparatus & materials	Activities	Evaluation
Problem (a) What is a Drug?	Drugs like Aspirin Antibiotic may be Displayed	A drug may be defined as a chemical substance which affects the living species mentally or physically.	Let the workers define a drug.
Problem (b) What are major categories of drugs?		Tell the workers that there are six major categories of drugs: 1) Tranquillizers 2) Narcotics 3) Hallucinogens 4) Stimulants 5) Sedatives 6) Miscellaneous Define the above categories of drugs. For example, tranquillizers are drugs, which are used to induce calmness, reduce tension and anxiety These drugs are available in the form of coloured pills and capsules.	

Contents	Examples, Apparatus & materials	Activities	Evaluation
		Chronic abuse of these drugs may result in the development of physical and psychological dependence.	
		Generally, tranquillizers are prescribed for nervous tension.	
What do you mean by physical and psychological dependence?		Have the workers discuss the terms of physical and psychological dependence.	Have the workers discuss about causes of AIDS.
		Summarize the state of physical dependence as a state of adaptation to a drug such that signs and symptoms of bodily discomfort appear when the drug is withdrawn abruptly.	
		Also, summarize psychological dependence as a strong emotional or mental drive to take a drug, either to obtain pleasure or avoid discomfort.	
What are ill effects of Using drugs intravenously?		Drug addicts, especially those using drugs intravenously, can be affected with HIV infection leading to a disease called AIDS (Acquired Immune Deficiency Syndrome).	

Contents	Examples, Apparatus & materials	Activities	Evaluation
Problem (c) What are medicinal uses and abuses of the following drugs? (1) Tranquilizer (2) Narcotics Drugs like: (A) Morphine (M, Mary, Whil Mojo)		**Excessive use may cause following side effects:** Headache, skin rashes, stomach disturbances, urinary frequency, withdrawal symptoms including insomnia, vomiting, shivering, loss of appetite, lack of muscular co-ordination, fever and occasionally, death. This drug when taken with alcohol can produce harmful effects. The most frequent tranquillizers diverted into illicit trade are maprobamate (Equanil, Miltown) and glutethimide (Doriden). Tell the workers that natural and synthetic morphine like drugs are the most effective pain relievers. Morphine is available as a fluffy, white powder found in cubes or tablets and is extremely bitter. These may be eaten or injected under the skin or intravenously. These drugs produce a sense of euphoria—an exaggerated sense of well being—drowsiness, nausea and urinary retention. In severe cases, the user may go into a coma. Death results when the individual can no longer breathe.	Have the workers discus in short the hazardous effects of tranquillizers.

Contents	Examples, Apparatus & materials	Activities	Evaluation
		Morphine users are generally lethargic and indifferent to their environment and personal situation. Hazardous effects of morphine are physical and psychological dependence, painful withdrawal symptoms, danger of acquiring hepatitis from contaminated needless and death from overdose.	Have the workers discuss hazardous effects of Narcotics.
(B) Heroin (H stuff, Junk Horse, Smack, Harry, Dynamite).		Heroin is available as a white crystalline powder, slightly bitter. May be sniffed, rarely taken by mouth or injected under the skin or intravenously. Signs and symptoms and hazardous effects are the same as those of morphine.	Have the workers discuss about causes of AIDS.
(C) Codeine		Tell the workers that codeine is approximately one-tenth as toxic as morphine. Codeine is usually available in the form of tablets or in cough syrups. Signs and symptoms and hazardous effects are same as those of morphine but milder.	

Contents	Examples, Apparatus & materials	Activities	Evaluation
(D) Hallucinogens		Tell the workers that hallucinogens are drugs which cause hallucinations. These drugs produce distortion of perception or dream images. These are called psychedelics.	Have the workers discuss an operational definition of "Psycedelics".
(3) Toxic solvents such as: (a) glue, nail polish remover, gasoline		Tell the workers that frequent use of toxic solvents produces psychological dependence, dizziness, headache, nausea, slurred speech and blurred vision and feelings of euphoria. Harm may be done to the brain, liver and kidney; and death due to suffocation is possible. Users generally have sweetish, sickly odour in breath and clothing.	Have the workers discuss in short "Toxic Solvents" and "Marijuana".
(B) Marijuana (Cannabis, Pot, Mary, Jane, Tea, Weedgrass, May Warmer, Rope Hempjive).		Marijuana is made of brownish green dried and shredded leaves with a pungent smell. It is smoked in a type of pipe or inhaler or as cigarettes. Discuss with the workers indicating that massive doses of marijuana may cause altered awareness of time and space, visual distortions and hallucinations. Mood changes ranging from anxiety to euphoria.	

Contents	Examples, Apparatus & materials	Activities	Evaluation
(C) Hashish (Hash)		Tell the workers that Hashish is available as a dark amber resinous material extracted from the flowering tops of the cannabis plant. It is smoked in a pipe or in a cigarette. Symptoms and hazardous effects are the same as those of Marijuana.	
(D) LSD (dLysergic acid diethylamide) common names: Acid, the Chief, the Hawk, the Cube, Big oz, Orange, Wedge, Sugar, 4-way, Big-" A".		Tell the workers that LSD was synthesized in 1938 from lysergic acid present in fungi that grow on rye and is available in the form of white powder or tablets or liquids or soaked in sugar cubes, clothing or blotting paper. LSD primarily affects the central nervous system producing changes in mood and behaviour. Hazardous effects involve physical and psychological dependence, extremely horrifying hallucination (bad trip or bum trip). Use of LSD may lead to chromosome damage and birth defects and suicidal urge.	

Contents	Examples, Apparatus & materials	Activities	Evaluation
(E) Mescaline common names: Mescal, Buttons, Peyote, Cactus		Inform the workers that mescaline is obtained from the Mexican cactus anhalonium. It is available in the form of gelatin capsules or in a form to be mixed with water or injected intravenously. Hazardous effects and symptoms are the same as those for LSD.	
(F) STP (Serenity		Tell the workers that STP is available in the form of blue or orange capsules or tablets which are swallowed. The peak effects occur three to five hours after being taken. Dryness of mouth, nausea, restlessness, dilated pupils are common symptoms.	
(4) Stimulants		Visual hallucinations, visual distortions, and change of mood may occur similar to those of LSD. Tell the workers that stimulants act on the central nervous system. Examples of stimulants are coffee, tea, cola. The synthetic stimulants are amphetamine and cocaine.	

Contents	Examples, Apparatus & materials	Activities	Evaluation
(A) Amphetamines common names: Speed Benne, Peppils, Ups, Dexies, Copilots, Footballs, Crystal.		Amphetamines are white, odorless, water soluble, bitter powder or volatile colourless liquid with a strong odour. Amphetamines may be sniffed, taken orally, or injected. Large doses produce fever, heart irregularities, convulsions or coma. Death may result from circulatory collapse. Amphetamines may also produce euphoria, insomnia, loss of weight, compulsion to talk and paranoid behavior.	
(5) Sedatives Barbiturates "Goofballs".		Tell the workers that sedatives have a depressant effect on the nervous system. The most commonly abused drug is "Barbiturates" or the street term is "goof ball". It is available in the form of pills, capsules, and injectable preparations. Hazardous effects are incoherency, intoxication, staggering gait, slurred speech, vomiting, drowsiness and depression. Large doses may produce	

		tremors, anxiety, delirium, convulsions, coma and death. Inform the workers that stramonium is available as a brownish-green powder. It is taken by inhaling the smoke of the powder when burned, or by swallowing. Dryness of mucous membrane, burning in throat, difficulty in swallowing, skin rash, rapid heart rate and convulsions are the common signs and symptoms. Activity No.1 Have the workers request for the information on drug use and abuse. The World Health Organization local health unit and state department on health services are reliable sources. Arrange a film about drug abuse and let the workers discuss it in the community. Activity No. II Invite persons with professional experience in drug abuse problems and request them to speak on the uses and abuses of drugs. Invite someone, who has been an addict or has	
(6) Miscellaneous Streamonium			(Al The workers will be evaluated on their active participation

Contents	Examples, Apparatus & materials	Activities	Evaluation
		Field Trip	
		Have the workers compile a list of community agencies concerned with drugs abuse, and arrange a field trip to some of those agencies.	
		States of U.P. Rajasthan and dry zones of eastern states produce the raw materials. Chemical processing yields narcotic properties. The triangular zone comprising India-PakistanNepal, S. East Asia is known as the Drug Pushing Zone.	
		The counselor may point out that the problems arising from alcohol are more dangerous than those from drugs.	
Problem (d) what are abuses of alcohol?		The workers may be told clearly and emphatically that when we drink alcohol, it means we put a drug into our system, which may produce damage to the digestive track, kidneys and liver. It may also produce impaired memory, chronic un-coordination and malnutrition.	

Contents	Examples, Apparatus & materials	Activities	Evaluation
Problem (d) What are abuses of alcohol?		There are three types of drinkers: (i) Casual (ii) Habitual (iii) Addicted The counselor may define the above terms in the following manner: Casual drinker is a person who drinks sometimes, and not because of overwhelming craving.	
What are the different types of drinkers?		A habitual drinker is a person who drinks regularly because of increasing dependence on alcohol i.e. on wine, beer or hard liquor. We may say that a habitual drinker is dependent on alcohol. Addicted drinker is one, who becomes a compulsive drinker. Drinking means everything to him.	Ask the workers to discuss about the three different stages of drinkers, i.e. Casual, habitual and addicted.
		The counselor may discuss the following signals of an alcoholic	The workers are asked to summarize the danger signals of an alcoholic.

Contents	Examples, Apparatus & materials	Activities	Evaluation
	Problem (e) What are the danger signals of becoming addicted to alcohol	—Drinking excessively—Craving for a drink in the morning or when depressed—Gulping drinks—Feelings of guilt—Blackouts— Hangovers— Hallucinations—Physical tremors—Badtemper	
		Let the counselor explain to the workers, the mechanism of alcohol absorption in the human system. For example, alcohol gets absorbed into our bloodstream through walls of the stomach and the small intestine.	The workers are required to discuss about the mechanism of alcohol absorption in the body. They may be evaluated with reference to their participatian.
	Problem (f) What happens to our system when we drink alcohol?	When absorbed, it is distributed throughout the body fluids. The rate of absorption depends on the amount of alcohol present in the system. About 95 per cent of the alcohol absorbed is utilized by the liver. The rest is eliminated through the urine. The liver can handle only a limited amount at a time (approximately one drink per hour). When the lever cannot burn excessive alcohol, the remaining alcohol stays in the system	

Problem (e) What are the danger signals of becoming addicted to alcohol?

and interferes with the functions of the central nervous system, resulting in embarrassing behavior, temporary loss of memory and nausea. The counselor may point out that excessive drinking may lead to the following disorders in the human system:

Problem (g) What are the long term effects of alcohol?s

(i)   digestive track disorders

(ii) cardiovascular disorders

(iii) kidney disorders

(iv) impaired memory

Problem (f) What happens to our system when we drink alcohol?

(v)   chronic uncoordination

(vi) sexual impotence

(vii) malnutrition

Problem (h) How does drinking alcohol affect driving?

(viii) physical dependence which may result in withdrawal symptoms such as nausea, anxiety, confusion, sweating, and vomiting

(ix) psychological dependence which may result in depression and boredom.

The counselor may invite a local doctor or a local health unit official, to discuss the long-term effects of alcohol, in

The workers are asked to discuss the long term effects of alcohol. They are evaluated on the basis of their active participation in the group.

detail. If possible, a film
on alcoholism alcoholism
may be shown. The
consuelor may mention
the following facts:

Alcohol affects the
reflexes immediately.

Alcohol narrows the
peripheral vision.
The average person is
impaired with a 0.5 per
cent blood alcohol level.

The workers are asked
to discuss their views
about the effects of
drinking while driving an
automobile.

It is an offence to drive
a vehicle with blood
alcohol level of over 0.08
percent.

The blood alcohol level
of a person weighing
150 Ibs and having 5
ounces of hard liquor
or 3.5 bottles of beer
could exceed 10 per cent.
The counselor should
emphasize that the only
safe policy is not to drink
at all, if driving.

Make the workers discuss
the abuses of alcohol
with their friends.

Films on Drug Education
and Alcohol.

Counselor may arrange
films on drug and
alcohol abuse.

		Let the workers discuss their opinions about the effects of drinking while driving an automobile. Let them discuss the issue with alcoholic parents or their friends. Screen the films on de-addiction of drugs and alcohol. Let the counselor take the workers for a demonstration at a local hospital for meaningful dialogue with physicians about the de-addiction.	The workers may be evaluated from a report about the film. The workers may be evaluated on their reports and discussion with alcoholics and de-addiction specialists.

CHAPTER 6

Some Practical Strategies for Preventing AIDS Among Young Industrial Workers

Poverty. They don't have anything.
They have no-one. They have nothing.
They are street cases . . .
We want the poor to feel loved.
We cannot go to them with sad faces.
God loves a cheerful giver.
He gives most who gives with joy.

Mother Teresa

We are all aware that the AIDS time-bomb is ticking and it may explode any time especially involving young industrial workers who could be the potential victims of this killer disease. It is also realized that the only method for preventing AIDS is through education i.e., bringing awareness and preventive strategies of this killer disease.

Thus it is of paramount importance to set up non-formal counseling centers for awareness and prevention of AIDS/HIV infection in every industrial unit.

(A) Establishment of non-formal counseling centers for awareness and prevention of AIDS/HIV infections in every industrial unit.

The environment in these non formal counseling centers should be that of friendship, i.e. an industrial worker develops friendly and cordial relationship with a counselor of the non-formal center, who should interact with HIV positive/AIDS victim/industrial workers with love and care. These non-formal counselors should be trained by AIDS experts. The preventive AIDS material should be developed in a very simple language.

The material may include frank, honest and straight forward talks about AIDS, meaningful messages regarding AIDS, posters, flip charts, audio-visual material and very light reading material in the form of comic books. All such material explaining the transmission and prevention of AIDS, should emphasize a positive attitude, hope, emotional and moral support to the persons who have already been infected with HIV virus.

The majority of industrial workers have been at a disadvantage because of lack of adequate education. Thus the orientation program for AIDS/ HIV infection prevention program should provide a feeling of self-esteem, motivation and an aim to live purposefully.

If these orientation programmes regarding AIDS prevention become fun and a pleasant activity, word is likely to spread soon about the useful information being imparted at such centers.

The course material in these programmes may include the following: knowing self, lifestyles, attitudes, aspirations, and expectations of young industrial workers, values clarifications problems of life and their possible solutions; sexually transmitted disease and AIDS, positive health care, family and community care.

In addition to the above activities, on holidays, an experiment in social living camps may be organized for these young industrial workers.

The main purpose of these camps should be to share experiences of life with reference to healthy living and prevention of AIDS in a relaxed and cordial atmosphere. The activities in these camps may include games and sports, cultural shows/street plays, exhibition regarding facts of life, positive health care, STD, AIDS and drug addiction etc. Such activities would make the industrial worker feel THAT he is "somebody" and boost his hope for the future with a feeling that he has a place in the economic and social life around him.

(B) Importance of values Clarification and Prevention of AIDS

As we are aware that the major cause of contracting AIDS is through indulgence in unsafe sex. It is also an admitted fact that emphasis should be given on the dynamics of "love making" with reference to sex. Love and sex are inseparable components of human nature, which is to be taken as a universal human value that includes respect for the other sex, compassion, sincerity and loyalty for each other Mahatma Gandhi's concept of love is very appropriate in this context, which suggests that when we say we love someone, we are supposed to respect that person i.e. his feelings, sentiments and values. There is no love when there is no respect. Concept of love has been aptly described by Late Krishnamurti, reputed International Spiritual leader:

"You do not say, '1 love the whole world, but when you know how to love one, you know how to love all, and love of humanity is factitious. When you love, there is neither one nor many, only love."

Maslow describes love as a part of being human. "The need for love characterizes every human being that is born."

Montague defines love as "one's needs are satisfied by persons whom one loves".

Thus if we can make our industrial workers understand the concept of sex in terms of "Love" as a basic human value the problem of AIDS/HIV infection through sex medium may be reduced.

Many of these young workers move to the environs of hostile urban cities, leaving behind the safe and protected life in their rural communities. Life in small towns in joint families is a well defined pattern. 'Right' and 'Wrong' are well treaded paths laid out by generations of 'Beliefs' held by orthodox communities. You learn to act in your watchful communities as you are expected to or face the wrath of elders, the 'panchayat' and the whole village. Even to this day in India the "powers" that the community has on individuals actions is nothing less than the dictates of royalty.

Therefore when young workers arrive in cities looking for jobs, the freedom and responsibility to take their own decisions about 'right' and 'wrong' is something beyond their training and capabilities. The struggle for survival and the confusion of making choices (the right ones) is too stressful for many. The cultural shock of the relative permissiveness in urban cities is absorbed by abandoning the traditional values and adopting the 'progressive' modern values promoted by TV, films, media and the city life itself. In the Process the young workers can fall pray to drug peddlers, pickpocket gangs, pimps and unhealthy sexual relationships. The transit populace and the workers in cities are at an enormous risk of contracting all kinds of diseases of which HIV/AIDS can be the worst because it destroys their ability to fight many common infections.

The urgent need to deal with the value crisis among the migrant youth should form part of the agenda of the industrial employers for workers orientation programme. Amalgamation of the best ideas of our traditional values with the practical enlightened approach of the modern ways could save our youth from the pitfalls of self destructive adoption of alien values.

A promising approach for dealing with the emerging value crisis among the youth, is the rejection of the Ideas of Imposing the right "values" upon them. Instead, one can teach them a process and a set of criteria by which they can themselves evaluate the soundness of their values. This approach might give the youth a set of tools and skills for sorting out the alternatives, which are available, and the consequences if they continue to live with a focus on their values.

Evidently both our society and its values are rapidly changing. The modern youth questions the values of his parents, teachers and leaders. If one is to cope with these changing attitudes, it is imperative to discuss the importance of values in the changing scenario. Values are acquired by examples and transmitted by what we do, not by what we say we should do. If we do not accept the concept of sex in terms of "love as a value", especially with reference to safe sex, it may be futile to discuss or preach the same to our modern generation. If we are to develop a process of assessing values, we must understand the background and environment of the youth. We need to provide them with opportunities to test their values. Errors in judgement may be discussed. But the older generation must be prepared to accept the values that the youth derive from the modern situations. The following strategies for value clarification may be quite helpful in overcoming the "value crisis" with special reference to sex issues.

These may include, My favourite activities, Discouraging apathy, Comparing values, Rating values, on the spot decisions, I am proud, In the public life, What am I ?, Chapter of my life, Picture of my life and Communication lines etc. which have been discussed in detail in the preceding chapters.

It has been found quite useful in group dynamics situations, especially during sex and love as a value in AIDS/HIV infection seminars.

CHAPTER 7

Clarification of Values and AIDS

You cannot teach a man anything,
You can only help him to find it within himself.

Galileo

As pointed out earlier, value conflict among the workers may lead to frustrations, and a feeling of helplessness, thus enticing them to alcohol and drug addiction, which could further lead to AIDS/HIV infection. It is also well known that values are acquired by examples of others and are transmitted by what we do, rather than by what we say we should do. If we had to develop a process for assessing values, we must understand the background and environment of our workers. We should provide them with equal opportunities to test their values. Errors in judgment must be discussed, but we must be prepared to accept the values the workers derive from the environment. Clarification of values is very important for alcohol, drug and sex.

However, the counselors of non-formal centers should be taught how to use various strategies for assessing values. Since most of industrial workers may not have adequate (Reading/Writing) skills, it may be desirable to have verbal discussions about these activities. Activities mentioned in this chapter are only suggestive in nature and not prescriptive. Counselor of the proposed non formal centers is the best judge to delete, modify, adopt or adapt these activities in the light of socio-economic and educational background of these industrial workers.

A.   Towards Values (Practical Strategies)

Sometimes in our routine, we ask a pertinent question, What am I doing here? No one knows the answer; people just make obvious guesses. Different religions give different answers, but an individual must decide for himself. Unless his life has a meaning, he won't have peace of mind. For this, he must have a set of values. By assigning certain values to his behavior in achieving the utmost goals, he can find a direction for his life.

Strategy No.1—My Favourite Activities

It aids the person in examining his favourite activities. By thinking about what you want to do, you will get a better idea of life. Once you decide upon such a goal, half the battle is won. This exercise is especially relevant for addicts.

Exercise: Discuss fifteen things you would like to do. These do not have to be important things; just anything you really enjoy doing. Think about what factor is involved in each such activity. Now examine your list, the counselor may help.

Strategy No.2—Discouraging Apathy

It will help the industrial workers to develop a stronger and clearer point of view.

Exercise: Take an important issue like AIDS prevention. Describe your views about it in a few words. Now ask these questions yourself: (Because of low illiteracy level the counselor may assist the industrial workers in this exercise and initiate discussions).

(1) What is your opinion about the following:

   (a) Pre-marital sex
   (b) Casual and unprotected sex
   (c) Safe Sex

(2) Are you confident of your position?
(3) Have you told someone about your stand on the issues?
(4) Any alternatives in making your decision?

(5) Have you analyzed the pros and cons of the issues and its aftermath?

(6) Is your stand based on your free choice?

(7) Anything about how you feel?

(8) Whether you feel the same when mentioned frequently?

Discuss how you actually came to your position on the issue with another person. What questions have you answered in the negative?

Go for another issue and find out if you had similar opinion In a more orderly fashion. Is our position stronger or weaker?

Exercise: The counselor may have a ladder or series of steps drawn on the black board or on a paper. He/she reads a situation and you will mark the best step that shows the strength of your feelings for and against on the subject. When each worker slots himself on the ladder, you will get a better idea of where you stand in relation to others. Discuss with the person—a few steps away from you—why he is more or less concerned about the issue than you are. Another way to gauge things is to test about five or six workers and rate each of them according to the strength of his feelings. These may be discussed orally by the counselors.

Example

Love her immensely	1
Love her without intimate relations	2
I will have intimate relations if she does not mind	3
I will not have sex without precautions	4
I will not have sex before marriage	5
I will not hurt her	6
I care for her	7
I respect her	8
I like her, she is just a friend	9

Strategy No. 4—In Between Issues

Answers do not remain concrete or practical in evaluation. You might have feelings somewhere in the middle. It gives you an opportunity to appreciate where you are undecided.

Exercise: An issue with two extreme options is presented to the group. Where are you? When you are called upon, briefly state your views (not reasons) on the issue and where you would put yourself on the line. Listen to others, you can discuss with appropriate reasons for your position. Did you end up in the middle or near one of the extremes? Where have the others ended up? Do you think you have average opinion on the subject or is it so important for you?

Think about:

1. How much freedom you have?
   I have no say . . . complete freedom.
   1 .10

2. Do you love your girlfriend?
   Just company . . . love her immensely

3. What is the nature of your relationship with your girl friend/boy friend?
   Physical pleasure . . . Friendship . . . Do not care about precautions . . .

4. How are your relations with your parents?
   Poor Satisfactory Good Very Good Excellent
   1-2 . . . 3-5 . . . 6-7 . . . 8-9 . . . 10 . . .

Strategy No.5—On the Spot Decisions

This exercise helps you in making quick decisions. It also serves as a quick method for people to gauge what others are thinking and how they react to questions.

Exercise: A question is put to you. Think carefully about it. Organize your thoughts so that you can state them briefly. Listen to others, who are called upon to speak.

Sample questions:

1. What issues have you spoken about recently in public?
2. What latest incident in the news has really upset you?
3. What issues in your community peeve you most?

Strategy No.6—I am Proud

It builds self-confidence in the worker and gives an idea about the degree of pride he has in the things he attempts to do.

Exercise: You are asked about your pride in relation to certain aspects of life. Do not compare your answers with those of other workers, but do try to get new ideas from them. Answer the question with the phrase, "I am proud . . ." or what makes you think, what makes you really feel good about. Don't answer with something you think you should be proud of, but really aren't.

Think about:

1.) What can you independently do and find yourself proud of?
2.) Which things are you proud of in relation to personal wealth?
3.) What are you proud of in your relationships with co-workers?
4.) What are you proud of in respect of something you have written?
5.) What are you proud of that relates to your family.
6.) What new learning experiences do you feel proud of?
7.) What are you proud of, especially in loving someone?
8.) Are you proud of your sincere concern for your girl/boy friend?
9.) Do you contribute anything to your community about which you feel proud?

Strategy No.7—In the Public Eye

Here, the workers will have a chance to state his opinion about some issues in the classroom. It also motivates him to stick to what he has said about the evaluation.

Exercise: A volunteer has to be interviewed by the counselors as the interviewer. He is asked several times about his beliefs and feelings on certain issues. He may refuse to answer any question, but those he chooses to answer must be answered truthfully. He may end the event at any time by thanking the audience. The volunteer at the end of the interview may ask the interviewer any of the questions he was asked. The number of questions put to the interviewer should be limited so as not to shift the focus from the volunteer.

Sample interviews:

1.) If you had a choice of how old you could be, what age would you like to be?
2.) Do you smoke? Why?
3.) Do you take hard drugs? Why?
4.) Do you believe in dating?
5.) What is your opinion about intimate sex relationship?
6.) Do you believe in intimate relations with precautions?
7.) Is there someone in your life who you admire very much? Why?
8.) Is there anything you really believe in?
9.) Which two things in your environment would you like to change?
10.) Name one thing you would like to change about yourself?

Strategy No.8—Sharing Experience

This enables you to get to know one another through interviews. You can relate on a more intimate basis if your group does not exceed six workers.

Exercise: Form groups of four to five people with the persons volunteering to be interviewed. The comperer will regulate the interview by calling upon one of the group members to ask question. The interviewee may pass on any question he does not wish to answer. The comperer can ask a member about the reason for asking it. When the group runs short of questions or when the interviewee says, "Thank you for the interview", judge that the interview is over.

Remember while interviewing:

1. People never talk about their personal ideas about sex. You should respect someone, if he decides to pass a question.

2. Attempt on arguments or commence lively debates. These interviews are to help the people in expressing their feelings, whereas for others it will serve as a basis for reactions in a mature way.

    If you disagree with someone try to understand his position; don't try to negate his feelings.

    If the groups are small or and you have sufficient time, you may interview others in your group. This exercise is more likely to succeed, if anyone gets an opportunity to express his feelings.

Strategy No.9—Learning to Listen

Trying to form a system of values is much easier when you are in an encouraging and warm atmosphere. To generate such an atmosphere, counselors and workers must learn to respect one another's views. Everyone has a right to express his opinion provided this fact is realized by all participants industrial workers will be afraid to voice their opinions.

Exercise: It attempts to help you accept and assimilate different opinions without mobilizing others to change their minds.

Everyone completes the format as:

1.) Like to be with people who . . .
2.) I don't like to be with people who . . .

Get into groups of three, do discuss your answers. Each person in the group should concentrate on the other two for a period of five minutes. The interviewer then talks about what he had written down.

Note:

1.) Give the interviewer your full attention for entire five minutes or hear him till he speaks. As only such questions that relate to the subject. Don't go off the track.
2.) Make him feel comfortable. It is not easy to talk in front of other people. Acknowledging his statements with nods or smiles will make everyone feel more relaxed. If you disagree with his statement try

not to show it. Negative feelings defeat the purpose of the activity. There will be discussion time later.

3.) Try to understand the other person's feelings. Ask a question to clarify the reason for a particular response. Make sure you are not trying to put yourself in the spotlight. Don't reveal any negative feelings through your questions.

4.) Think about how well you have listened and understood them. Did you have a hard time saying nothing when someone was commenting on the subject you disagreed with? Were you afraid of giving your opinion? Discuss and react to each other's positions for another five or ten minutes. Did you feel more confident or less confident than before? Could you listen to them as well, by knowing that you could say something this time?

Strategy No.10—Examining Alternatives

How many times have you committed and found yourself regretting it afterwards? May be, if you had been more clear about your feelings you could have reacted in a more beneficial way. This strategy will help you in conditioning the alternatives before taking any decision. The purpose here is to motivate a pupil in accordance with his/her personal values.

Let us discuss the thing you have done that you regretted later. Now in a situation where something must be done, decide what alternative is the best. Assimilate all your feelings related to the situation and your role in this situation. Answer one: you think, you would probably do, and the second: you think, you should do. Break into groups of three or four for discussion and arrive at a conclusion.

Exercise: Suppose a girl in your neighborhoods is pregnant before marriage—discuss the issue.

Strategy No. 11—Discussion with Self

How do you spend your time and money? Do you spend it wisely? These things are important for us to know it we want to move from where we are to what we ought to be in life. This strategy also makes you examine how you live through your life.

The counselor may draw a circle on a paper and divide it into four quarters. Each quarter represents six hours of the day. Now try to estimate how much time you spend on each of these things.

1.) Sleeping
2.) Working
3.) Working for welfare of your community
4.) With your colleagues
5.) Doing something by yourself
6.) Doing nothing
7.) Helping in community services such as drug de-addiction, hygiene and AIDS prevention awareness.
8.) With your family including sharing meals
9.) On other things

You won't get exact estimates, but have to add up to 24 hours—to call it a routine.

1.) Think about:
2.) Are you happy with the size of your slices?
3.) Draw another apple you think would be perfect. Is it very different from the first?

Anything feasible you can do to change the sizes of your slices?

Strategy No.12—Make a Wish

Exercise: Let us assume that we have a magic box. It has everything that you can possibly want, tangible or intangible within. If you had such a box in front of you right now, what could have been stored in it? Take your own time with the correct answer, then jot it down.

Is your answer related to money?
Is your answer related to vi rtue?
Do you think your answer will change In the next year, month or week, tomorrow?
What do you want for a friend?
What do you want for a favorite relative?
What do you want for society?

What do you want for the world?
Keep your answers; look at them sometime again in the next week.
See whether your values have changed.

Strategy No.13—What Am I?

Exercise: This strategy will help you to acquaint yourself better with personality development. It will give you opportunity to think about your life objectively.

Write a short story once in two or three days.

Use the topics?

1.) What am I?
2.) What do I want to be?
3.) I feel proud . . .
4.) My most valuable experience
5.) A turning point
6.) If I were the President of my country
7.) My best friend
8.) My best teachers.

You may discuss your stories or read them aloud.

Strategy No.14—My Life

This activity will help you to see your life as a whole. It gives you an opportunity to think of goals—past and present and not living through the days as they come. It will help you to be more confident of the pattern of your life and the way you change it to suit you better.

During the years, you will develop chapters or pages for your life story by remembering the past events. Examine such experiences to unveil important life partners and whether these were results of conscious choice, outside pressures or impulses. Discuss a page or two with someone frequently. Learn about their experiences and feelings about them.

Examples

1.) Who have been your favourite teachers—not only school teachers but anyone who might have taught a valuable lesson to you especially regarding life skills?
2.) Draw a line with one end representing birth and the other, your age now. Mark all the turning points in your life on it. Put your age underneath each mark, representing the turning points. How did they happen? How did you feel about these before and after? Did anyone notice the sudden change? How do you feel about it now?
3.) Write episodes about some of the learning experiences.—Learning to ride a bike. Who helped? Whose bike was it?

> ➤ Learning to dance—learning to play cards
> ➤ Learning to love your brothers and sisters
> ➤ Learning to respect your next door girl
> ➤ Any other experience you have had, including the use of narcotic drugs especially with syringe and having sex without condoms.

Strategy No.15—Picture of my life

This strategy helps the workers to think about the direction to their lives. How important it is and why they want to change?

Exercise:

1.) What is the most important thing you have done in your life?
2.) What is the most important thing your family has done?
3.) What is it that someone can do to make you happy?
4.) What do you want to achieve with only one year at your disposal?
5.) What was your greatest personal failure?
6.) Which thing would you do to prevent AIDS/HIV infection in your community?

Break into discussion groups and compare your notes. Explain the reasons and listen to comments from others. Do you think your answers will change by next year? How do you like to change? In which direction is your life moving? Are you being moulded by other or do you control yourself in the building of your character?

Strategy No.16—Communication Lines

Many feelings in our world are lost or wasted, because people can't communicate smoothly. They are rather worried about what they are about to say next when they miss the valuable point of others. Building values comes from considering alternatives. The latter comes from listening to the opinions of other people. By listening and feeling we can completely understand their opinions. This is not an easy thing i.e. listening with rapt attention to someone you disagree with. It helps in the long run, when it comes to investigating fully each alternative before making any decision. Understanding people better can also make life less complicated. Exercise: Break into groups of four with one person acting as the monitor and the others as participants. The monitor introduces an issue, such as sex education in schools, on which the others have different opinions. When each person makes his statement, the next person must repeat the point he made before giving his opinion. Each person must be satisfied about his opinion being heard before someone else speaks. The discussion winds up when everyone gets exhausted over the topic. A brief discussion may follow with the whole group. How well did you listen? Did you interpret the opinions of other persons? Were you satisfied with the attention you had? Did you feel happy about your opinion?

To conclude, the counselor in the non-formal centers may conduct these activities regarding values clarification among young industrial workers in a very simple manner. We are all aware that literacy level of most young industrial workers is not very high. More emphasis has to be given on verbal discussions.

CHAPTER 8

Healthy Living
(A Curriculum Unit for the Counselors)

He who postpones the hour of living rightly is like the rustic who waits for the river to run out before he crosses.

Haraco Epitles L.,

The unit discusses the importance to understand physiology of our body and its development. To impart this knowledge to the workers, is of great importance, as among the less fortunate people there are many unhealthy and un-hygienic habits. The workers should be made to understand that eating is one of the most enjoyable activities for body development. Choice of food determines the vitality, health and appearance of a man. Thus food has more values than just to provide a pleasant tastes. Failure in eating a proper and balanced diet leads to disorders in the Human body. (Most of the workers, are undernourished or they do not eat the right food). The counselor should discuss the importance of a balanced diet and good living habits and harms caused by eating spoiled food. Spoiled vegetables are sold at very low rates in India. Due to poverty, poor people buy these spoiled vegetables without caring for the damage they may cause the body.

The counselor should discuss about the nature of patent medicines without going much into the technical detail. In every community, there are so many unqualified doctors (quacks, without having any proper medical knowledge. Sometimes these home-made medicines could prove fatal. The workers should be made aware of disadvantages of the medicines prescribed by quacks. Many medicines that seem to "cure" could cause irreparable damage in the long run.

Contents	Examples, Apparatus & materials	Activities	Evaluation
Problem I: What is Food?		Have the workers discuss definition of food and aid the workers in arriving at a conclusion that food is a chemical substance which provides materials for body growth. Give a lecture on the essential ingredients of our food. The counselor should explain the fact that the body tissues are largely protein in character, so their growth and replacement requires foods containing similar materials. The workers are required to discuss importance of proteins in our food It means that protein must be contained in some of the foods we eat. Young people should take food rich in proteins e.g. milk, eggs, cheese. Also tell the workers that carbohydrates are the source of energy.	The workers are required to discuss the importance of proteins in our food.

Contents	Examples, Apparatus & materials	Activities	Evaluation
		If possible, arrange to have some common vitamins, for example: Vitamin A Tablets. Vitamin C Tablets: multivitamins and calcium etc.	
		Give a lecture on the role of vitamins in our food.	
		Give a definition of vitamins as organic compounds found in certain foods. Explain they have a regulatory action in the human body.	The workers are required to discuss the foods and the vitamins they contain.
		The workers are required to discuss the foods and the Vitamins they contain.	
Problem II: What are Vitamins?		Give a lecture on the role of vitamins in our food. Also explain the effect of lack vitamins in our food. Provide a table which lists the important vitamins and shows their relation to health.	
		Tell the workers that the human body cannot create any chemical element it can only recombine elements supplied by Food.	Why should we take a balanced diet?

Contents	Examples, Apparatus & materials	Activities	Evaluation
Problem III: What is a balanced diet?		Emphasize the fact that in order to assure ourselves of the necessary food materials. We should eat what is called a balanced diet. The counselor should exhibit pictures illustrating various diseases (rickets, bone malformation) due to unbalanced diet.	
		Standard balanced diet table in terms of calories (It can be obtained from a government hospital)	
	Standard balanced diet table in terms of calories (it can be obtained from a government hospital)	Emphasize the fact that eating is not only one of the most enjoyable activities but is also one of the most essential activities for a body's development. Failure to eat a proper and balanced diet is to invite diseases in the human body.	
	Sugar (Gur) Coke (Soda Water)	Provide a sample of balanced diet. Have the workers discuss the food that they eat with regard to the calorie content.	The workers will be evaluated from the participation in the group activities.
		Give a lecture on the harmful effects of undesirable food; e.g.spoiled vegetables which are sold at lower price can produce harmful effects in our body.	Ask the workers to take their two days food list & compare it with the list of food in terms of vitamins.

Contents	Examples, Apparatus & materials	Activities	Evaluation
		Most of us eat too much sugar (gur) Sugar has definitely undesirable effects. It increases the possibility oftooth decay and spoils the appetite for healthier food. Much of the sugar, in "soda water" (soft drink) is of doubtful value. Many of the flavours, the acid, and the colouring matter are synthetic coal tar chemicals or extracts from plants which are not considered to be foods. Too much of any acid increases the danger of tooth decay. Exhibit the pictures of rats or persons eating unbalanced diet or poor diet.	
Problem IV: What is the result of poor diet?	Pictures of rats or person eating poor diet	The workers are asked to discuss the results of poor diet. Give a lecture on the diseases caused by poor diet e.g. knock knees, bow legs, small lower jaws, twisted teeth, anemia. Invite a qualified doctor to explain the importance of a balanced diet, harmful effects of eating spoiled vegetables and about good living habits.	The workers are asked to discuss tke result of poor diet. The workers are asked to discuss "Good living habits" giving their own examples, especially from their homes.

Contents	Examples, Apparatus & materials	Activities	Evaluation
Problem V: What is the nature of patent medicines?	Some common potent medicines like Detol (antiseptic), Vitamin (tonic), Medicines prepared by unregistered medical practitioners.	Have workers list the patent medicines used in their homes. Exhibit some common patent medicines such as laxatives. Make the workers read the labels on some of the bottles and discuss their contents. Critically examine the homemade medicines given by unregistered medical parishioners and elicit the following: (a) These may contain harmful ingredients (b) Some are habit forming (c) Dosage recommended may not be correct as the doctor is unqualified. (d) The medicines might not have been prepared in a scientific manner (e) The preparation might be too old. Round Table Conference	The workers are asked to discuss the disadvantages of home made medicines.

		Have the workers discuss good living habits and the contributions of science in improving our daily life.	
		Arrange an exhibition on AIDS with supporting information.	
		Exhibition may include maximum posters, films regarding AIDS prevention & Alcohol, Drug addiction	
Summary Questions:			The workers will be evaluated from their active participation in the discussion.
What are good living habits?			
Problem VI What is AIDS?			

Conclusion: The Importance of a healthy way of Living is self evident but awareness about the harmful impact of eating, drinking and indulging in an unhealthy way has to be impressed upon the simple minds of many illiterate and less fortunate people.

CHAPTER 9

Community Awareness Drive in Education and Prevention of AIDS

Social justice is the best way to ensure sustainable peace and eradicate poverty. And I believe in people coming together organizing, joining their voices

Juan Somavia ILO Director General.

We are aware that the killer disease AIDS is attacking the developing countries in a big way, especially in Industrial sectors. This may affect our young industrial workers who become sexually active. It may also affect workers who are victims of social evils like alcohol and drug addictions (due to various reasons such as lack of meaningful education, poverty, frustration and absence of proper role models).

Generally, young industrial workers live in a cluster, a "bastee" or a "Chawl". This is a community where all people work or atleast under socially healthy conditions all should work. In these places there are many problems of sanitation, health, hygiene, water pollution, alcohol, drugs and sexual harassment etc. One of the burning issues in the community is how the community should be mobilized so that they do not become victim of alcohol, drug abuse, unsafe sex and AIDS. It is gratifying to note that recently a meaningful role is played by Panchayat in educational process especially in the rural and disadvantaged urban community. The role of trade unions in the industry in bringing awareness and preventing AIDS in this industrial community is very crucial and cannot be over emphasized. To deliberate upon the role of community, it is necessary to discuss the term "community power."

Role of Community Power Structure

Community Power is the ability of individuals or groups to determine the behavior of others, against their wishes. The structure of power within a community refers to the relationship between individuals and groups holding power.

For desired educational changes, with the initiation of prevention of AIDS and drug abuse programmes, the educators, administrators, professionals and local community leaders need to develop appropriate strategies in prevailing power structure, which may:

(i) promote the adoption of power structure, though the mobilization of community services, local advisory committees and the existing political structure in a community; and

(ii) produce an appreciable change to make it open to radical AIDS prevention and Drug addiction programmes among industrial workers and their families.

In the community comprising of Chawl, Bastee, where generally these industrial workers live, the above strategies can be materialized by the utilization of the services of local advisory committees and the community power structure.

Local community groups may comprise individuals and organization in the industrial communities who want to help in the prevention of AIDS educational programmes. These committees might include counselors of proposed non-formal centers, representatives from the respective industry, professional and local community people who are directly or indirectly concerned with and/or interested in prevention of AIDS and other related health education issues. This approach will ensure local public involvement in the welfare of the community. The concept of Local advisory committees for bringing awareness and prevention of HIV/AIDS is of great importance if the company management provides residential and medical facilities for their industrial workers

Local Advisory Committee

It would be worthwhile to deliberate upon the term 'Local Advisory Committee' (LAC) which may be conceived as a group of local community people as mentioned earlier whose function is to advise the industry management, trade union and the community members relating to prevention of AIDS programmes with special reference to alcohol, drugs and sex related matters in the context of our cultural, social and moral values. In order to ensure that the local advisory committees have a wholesome impact on the welfare of the local industrial community with special reference to prevention of AIDS among industrial workers, it is necessary to specify their advantages, organization, functions, and intent in the matters especially relating to AIDS education.

Advantages of LACs

(1) It enhances awareness regarding AIDS monster and its prevention among industrial workers.
(2) It provides a climate in the community which discourages some social evils among industrial workers. This may include indulgence in alcohol drug addiction and other socially undesirable practices prevalent in the local industrial community.
(3) It improves the quality of life among industrial workers with reference to healthy living habits.

The impression that the present day Indian society is dormant, static and impervious to social, economic and scientific changes is highly misleading. In spite of its 47.79 per cent illiteracy, the people have the wisdom of ages. They are cautious and not dazzled by appearances. Despite their well-tried, time-honoured, even primitive ways of doing things, they will make sure that the new ways will work. The society is not quiescent, but it's the concern for security which determines the attitude of change They all want welfare of the workers and try to overcome social evils i.e. alcohol, drug addiction, unhealthy living habits, and unsafe sex etc. What they want is new, relevant, meaningful and problem solving approach to these social evils and not merely novel in usage. If we want to prevent AIDS among young industrial workers, we must help them to meet the/felt needs. The system should seek the opinion and active involvement of community members to win their support for enriching the quality of life. This approach increases public understanding of AIDS problems and other problems relating to alcohol and drug abuse.

Local Advisory Committees as proposed above are established to give advise rather than for decision making. The meaning of "advisory" should be made very clear to the local advisory committee in order to avoid any possible future conflict over their magnitude of influence and power.

A local advisory committee may select its Chairman, Vice Chairman and Secretary. The Chairman may be a non-professional with a good reputation in the community, one who can feel the pulse of the community better.

Suggestions for LAC (Local Advisory CommiTTee)

(i)   The Local Advisory Committee should be aware of local as well as national interests while making any decisions.
(ii) It should have the ability to work with individuals and organizations with diametrically opposite views in a generally democratic and cooperative manner.
(iii) There should be clear methods of communication. In any suggestion for prevention of AIDS, drug and alcohol abuse educational programmes, the committee should be unanimously opined.
(iv) Organize a community fair on exhibition showing the methods of AIDS prevention. The after effects on the human physiology of drug and alcohol abuse may be exhibited through multimedia approach such as films, posters and lectures.

To implement the AIDS preventive educational program and to involve local community members in the local advisory committee, it may be imperative to orient them regarding AIDS preventive strategic drug and alcohol abuse.

CONCLUSION

The Imminent need to address the issues of prevention and treatment of HIV/AIDS among industrial workers is quite apparent. Without any further delay, special actions are imperative to control and check the HIV/AIDS Epidemic, because the impact of deprivation of industrial and transport workers will be tremendous on more privileged citizens if AIDS related programmes for them are not implemented on a war-footing. To sum up, we quote Dr. Peter Piot-UNAIDS Executive Director:

"Until we recognize AIDS as the Development and security issue of our time we cannot success in beating the Epidemic."

ANNEXURE I

General Information About Sex and HIV Infections

i.) By sexual intercourse during which the semen or vaginal fluid of an infected person passes into the body of another person. HIV can be passed in this way from man to man, man to woman, or woman to man. Worldwide, nine out of ten infections in adults have been passed on through sexual intercourse.

ii.) By the use of unsterilized needles or synnges for injecting drugs.

iii.) By blood transfusion if the blood used is (unknowingly) infected with H IV

iv.) By an infected woman to her unborn child.

— If a mother is infected with HIV, then there is a risk that she may give the virus to her baby. But where other diseases are a common cause of death in babies, breast feeding is not a great risk. Without safe water, sterilized bottles and tests, and milk powder, bottle-fed babies are much more likely to become malnourished, and to die, than babies who are breastfed. In such conditions, it is safer for the child to be breastfed even if the mother is infected with HIV.

— It is not possible to get HIV from being near to or touching someone infected with the virus. Hugging, shaking hands, coughing, sneezing will not spread the diseases. HIV cannot be transmitted through seats, telephones, plates, glasses, spoons, towels, bed-linen, swimming pools, or public baths.

— A person infected with HIV is not a public health danger. Any injection with an unsterilized needle or syringe is dangerous.
— A needle or syringe can pick up small amounts of blood from the person being injected. If that person's blood contains HIV and if the same needle or syringe is used for injecting another person without being sterilized then HIV can be transmitted
— Those who inject themselves with drugs are therefore particularly at risk from AIDS. So are people who have sex with those who inject drugs.

Drug injection is in itself dangerous. But because of the additional risk of HIY, those who don inject drugs should never use another person's needle or syringe or allow their own to be used by others.

— National Child Immunisation Programmes use needle which are sterilized between each use and are therefore, safe. All infants should be taken for a full course of immunizations in the first year of life.
— Other injections are often unnecessary, as many useful medicines can be taken by mouth. Where injections are necessary, they should be given only by a trained person using a sterilized or a disposable needle and syringe.
— Ear-piercing, dental treatment, tattoing, facial marking and acupuncture are not safe if the equipment used is not sterilized. It is also not safe to be shaved by a barber using an unsterilized razor.
— AIDS/HIV infection can be prevented through education as there is no cure or vaccine available for this killer disease. There are also aids/messages for woman/men which can obtained from UNICEF/WHO/UNESCO/UIDP or local hospitals.

AIDS is an incurable disease. It is caused by a virus which can be passed on by sexual intercourse, by infected blood, and by infected mothers to their unborn children.

➢ AIDS is caused by HIV virus known as the human immune deficiency virus (HIV). HIV damages the body's defence system. People who have AIDS die because their body can no longer resist the attack by micro-organisms of other serious illness.
➢ People infected with HIV usually go for many years with unnoticed signs of any disease. They may look and feel perfectly normal and

healthy during that period. But anybody infected with HIV can infect others.

➤ AIDS is the later stage of HIV infection. It takes on an average 7 or 10 years for AIDS to develop from the time when a person is first infected with HIY. AIDS is not curable, although some medicines have been developed to keep people with AIDS healthier for longer time.

➤ Anyone who suspects that he or she may have been infected with HIV should contact a health worker or an AIDS testing centre. It is vital for those who have the virus to learn how to avoid passing it to others, and to receive advice about how to take care of their own health.

➤ HIV can only be passed from one person to another in a limited number of ways.

ANNEXURE II

Useful Information for Counselors of Non-Formal Centers in the Industries (General slangs terms used by Drug Addicts)

L.S.D.

Acid—L.S.D.

Trip—L.S.D. Experience Acid Head—A person who is addicted to L.S. D.

Cube Head—Psychologically dependent on l.S.D.

Also called Acid Freak Electric Koolade—American soft drink produced synthetically with l.S.D.

Other slang terms for l.S.D.

Purple Haze, Sunshine, Pyramid, Big 0, the Big Chief, HeavenlySunshine, Window Pane, ete.

Hashish Air Plane—A hashish cigarette butt Pot head—Hash Addict

Other slang terms for Hashish Angel Dust, Charas, Mary Jane, Mexican Brown, Hemp, Hash, Shit, Pot, Dope

COCAINE Candy, Snow, Junk, Coke, Dust, Hard Stuff

HEROIN Smack, Horse, Harry, Hard Stuff, Joy Powder, Junk Scotch, Coballo (Spanish), Dope

MARIJUANA Bhang, Black Stuff (Opium)

MORPHINE Powder, Dreamer, Junk Morth, Dope

General Communication Terms used by Drug Addicts

Ball	—	Sexual Intercourse
Blast	—	Strong effect of drugs
Blast Party	—	Drug addicts party with music and sex
Boost	—	To steal, Rip off
Bread	—	Money
Busted	—	Arrested
Buzz	—	The drug feeling or sensation
Chick	—	Girl
Coked	—	Under the influence of cocaine
Cokie	—	Cocaine addict
Cop	—	Policemen
Creacke	—	Druugs peddler and physician
Cut	—	Adulterated drugs
Daisy	—	Dexedirine pills

Downers	—	Drugs that put you to sleep
Dynamit	—	Pure and high quality drugs
For out	—	Wonderful, Highly pleasurable experience
To fix	—	To inject
Flash	—	Effect of drug being injected in the vein
Flip	—	Psychotic
Flip Chick	—	Crazy girl
Freak	—	Drug addict
Freak-out	—	Enjoy under influence of drugs
Fuzz	—	Police
Gun	—	Syringe and needle
Hard Stuff	—	Heroin, Cocaine, Morphine
Head Shrinker	—	Psychiatrist
Heat	—	Feeling of sexual intercourse due to drugs
Hooked	—	Addicted
Junkie	—	Heroine or morephine addict
Nabbed	—	Arrested
Pad	—	Drugs addicts dwelling
Pusher	—	Drugs peddler

Queen	—	Male homosexual who assumes female role
Pothead	—	Hash addict
Pot Party	—	Pothead's get-together
Score	—	To buy
Shit	—	Drugs, mainly hash
Stoned	—	Under influence of drugs
Big Jo or Uncle	—	Policeman

ADDITIONAL SUGGESTED READINGS

➤ Ansi, Perakyla, AIDS Counselling, Institutional Interaction and Clinical Practice, Cambridge University Press, (1992).

➤ Anderson, Roy M& Robert May, "Understanding the AIDS Pandemic", Scientific America, May 57-62 (1971).

➤ Azima, Diet Pattern of working class families, Indian Workers, 29 Boardhan A.B. Developing many sided activities in workers colonies 30 (23), Bergel, Frank Dayies, All About Drugs, London: Nelson Publishers.

➤ Bhardwaj (Trans), Light of Truth, (Swami Dayanand Saraswati), S.A.PS. Publishers, New Delhi (1982).

➤ Champakala Lakshmi R. Working conditions of women young workers (i), p. 14.

➤ Chaudhari K.K, Perspectives on Indian Industrial Workers, Integrated Management, 14 (10-12), pp 30-36 (1992).

➤ Chitala Vineeta, Shanker Das and Vimla Nadkarni, A Study of knowledge Attitudes, Beliefs and Practices on AIDS in 4 locals in Maharashtra: A Report, Bombay: Tata Institute of Social Sciences.

➤ Chutani, C. Et. Al., Awareness and Knowledge about AIDS among Rural Population in India, "Care Calling", 3 (4) pp 20-22.

➤ Clemens, Alphonse H., Catholicism and sex", The Encyclopedia of Sexual Behaviour, New Your: Hawthorne Books Inc.

➤ Des, S.R. Mohan, T. Indian Labour Scene (a collection of essays). The author, Dhesi, Avtar Singh & M.S. Dhariwal, Health Education and Productivity of Industrial Worker, Amiritsar Margin 13 (2), pp 53-57.

➤ Dube, K.C. Drug abuse in Northern India", No 1.

➤ Encylopedia of Sexual Behaviour, New York, Howthorn Books, Inc Pp 440-155 Ganguli, H.C., Behavioural Research in Sexuality, Delhi: Vikahs Publishing House Pvt. Ltd, (1992).

➤ Gopalkrishanan, K., "Promoting Condoms", Seminar, 396; pp 34-36,.

➤ Jiloha, R.C. And Sain, B., Porm Drug to Dragon, New Delhi Mittal Publications Kakkar, S., Intimate Relations: Exploring Indian Sexuality", New Delhi, Penguin Books India Pvt. Ltd.

➤ Kalra, R.M. Drug Addiction in Schools (Revised), New Delhi, Vikas Publishing House, Kalra R.M., AIDS and Adoscents—A New Generation at Risk, New Delhi, Vikash Publishing House (1995).

➤ Kalra, R.M., Presenting AIDS I & II, Statesman, Feb. 22& 29.

➤ Kalra, R.M., Drug Addiction, Real Life must be Meaningful, Statesman, Nov. 14.

➤ Kalra, R.M. AIDS, Sexuality and Homosexuality:, New York:

➤ W.W., Nortorn and

➤ Jayasuriya, D.C. HIV Law and Law Reforms (Asia and Pacific), New Delhi: UNDP Regional Project on HIV and Development,

> Leech, Kenneth and Brenda Jordan, Drug for Young People—The Use and Misuse, Oxford:

> The Religious Education Press Ltd.

> Nag Moni, Sexual Behaviour and AIDS in India, Baltimore: John Hopkin Univ,—New Delhi, Vikas Publishing House Pvt. Ltd, 1996.

> NACO, Good of India, National AIDS Control Programme", India, Country Scenario: An Update, Delhi: Ministry of Helath and Family Welfare, (1991).

> McDermott Jim, "The AIDS Epidemic in Asia", Washington (D.C.): Task Force on International AIDS/HIV.

> Sain Bhim, "Drugs: Education as Weapon" in the Tribune, Chandigarh, 13 March Sharma Baldev R. The Indian Industrial Worker, Issues in Perspective, Vikas, p205 Youth and Drugs, a WHO Publication.

www.ingramcontent.com/pod-product-compliance
Lightning Source LLC
Chambersburg PA
CBHW031248280526
45784CB00004B/1766